Therapy in Acute Coronary Care

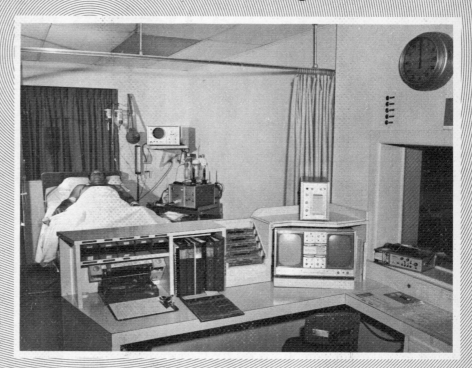

BARRY B. WHITE

THERAPY *in* ACUTE CORONARY CARE

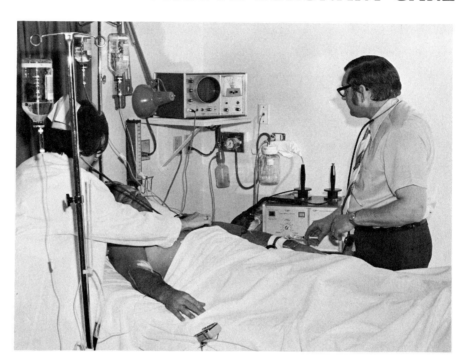

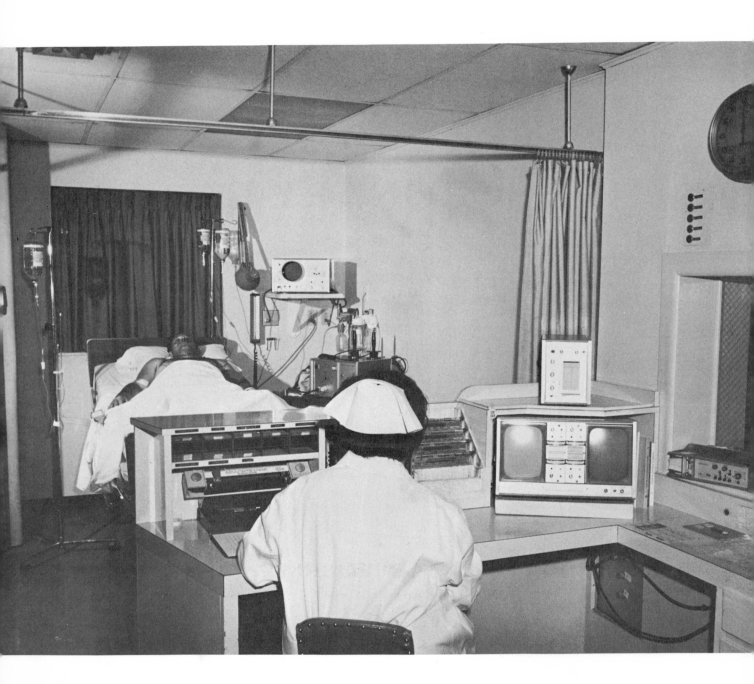

THERAPY
IN
ACUTE CORONARY CARE

BARRY B. WHITE, M.D.

McPheeters Clinic, Poplar Bluff, Missouri

YEAR BOOK MEDICAL PUBLISHERS · INC.

35 EAST WACKER DRIVE · CHICAGO

Library of Congress Catalog Card Number: 70-138938

International Standard Book Number: 0-8151-9275-4

NOTICE

Every effort has been made to be certain that the drug dosages herein are accurate and in accord with the standards acceptable at the time of publication. However, new discoveries know no timetable. Thus the author and publisher strongly urge the reader, especially with new and infrequently used drugs, to check the production information sheet included in the package of each drug he plans to use to be certain there are no changes in the recommended dosage or administration

Preface

When attempts were made to find a comprehensive reference source of therapy as applied to the patient with acute myocardial infarction cared for in the acute coronary care unit, it was found that a great deal of excellent information was available for the physician and nurse in the form of texts, manuals, booklets and articles; but that the information was not consolidated into one readily available reference source and, therefore, was not realistically accessible for ready reference to an individual not well versed in the literature of acute coronary care.

Since a majority of patients with acute myocardial infarction are cared for in small community hospitals, and frequently by nurses and physicians who have not had opportunity for extensive training in the care of acute myocardial infarction in the coronary care unit, it seemed a necessity that a manual on the special aspects of therapy of acute myocardial infarction as carried out in the coronary care unit be made available.

It became apparent that review of or learning the basics of normal physiology as well as pathologic physiology related to the cardiovascular system (and in particular the autonomic nervous system) was necessary for understanding the dynamics of therapy of acute myocardial infarction. This manual represents an attempt to compile, from numerous excellent reference sources, a basic outline of the *therapy of acute myocardial infarction in the coronary care unit*. Presentation is made in outline form to facilitate use of the manual.

It has been assumed, in assembling this manual, that the patient with acute myocardial infarction will be cared for in an acute coronary care unit by a staff of specially trained nurses. It is recognized that nurses in some coronary care units may have had more intensive specialized training than others, and it is hoped that this manual will be of aid both to the nurse who has and the one who has not had wide opportunity for specialized training.

Similarly, it is realized that all physicians caring for patients in the acute coronary care unit will not have had the specialized training of the cardiologist, and it is our hope to aid the physician who has not had a great deal of prior training in acute coronary care.

I wish to express my gratitude to Robert E. Kleiger, M.D. (Cardiologist; Director of the Medical Intensive Care Unit, Jewish Hospital of St. Louis; Assistant Professor of Medicine, Washington University School of Medicine) for his kindness and patience in reviewing the manuscript and his suggestions concerning change and improvement. My thanks to Miss Paralee Diamond and Mrs. Lena McPheeters for their understanding patience in the preparation of the manuscript in final form.

BARRY B. WHITE

Table of Contents

Introduction

This manual is intended for use by all personnel primarily responsible for the patient in the acute coronary care unit, including both physicians and nurses. Its utilization may vary—from that of a primary source of treatment information to use as a source of reference information. The uses will depend on the personnel utilizing the manual and the circumstances of use in the individual institution.

Intended Purpose for Physicians

The purpose of this manual for physicians is to review the generally accepted therapy of acute myocardial infarction, particularly as that therapy has been altered by the advent of the coronary care unit and by continuous electrocardiographic monitoring available to acute coronary care. An attempt has been made to bring together in concise form as much information as space will permit. Therefore the information is presented in outline form for ease of learning, review and reference. This manual is most specifically intended for physicians who have not had extensive experience in caring for patients in the acute coronary care unit.

Intended Purpose for Nurses

The purpose of this manual for nurses is to present information concerning therapeutic measures in the acute coronary care unit. This information is designed to be somewhat more advanced than that available in the basic instruction courses arranged for nurses preparing to begin their duties in the coronary care unit. Parts of the manual may also be suitable for teaching the basics of therapy to those preparing to begin their duties in the coronary care unit and as a reference source for pharmacologic agents and methods utilized in therapy.

It is assumed that nursing personnel utilizing this manual will have had, or are receiving, training regarding the specialized functions of the coronary care unit. Therefore no emphasis has been placed on the unit size, physical facilities, electronic equipment, staffing, specialized nursing role or the total nurse training program which must be taken into account in the initial planning for and staffing of a coronary care unit. It is also assumed that the nurse has learned, or is learning, to interpret electrocardiograms for the purposes of diagnosing arrhythmias. There are numerous excellent sources of such information in the literature.

Some procedural protocols are included in the Appendix. These are intended as representative samples. Each procedural protocol must ultimately be specifically established for the institution providing acute coronary care.

Certain sections of this manual contain material that might be considered too highly technical for adequate understanding or realistic utilization by the nurse. It is hoped that the manual is so designed that these sections may be omitted without detracting from its over-all value.

Discussion

The many facets of acute coronary care as carried out in the intensive coronary care unit have been well outlined by experienced clinicians in the literature over the past few years. Many excellent sources have presented information concerning the difficult task of establishing, organizing and operating these specialized intensive care units.[*] Numerous clinicians have reviewed the purposes and functions of the coronary care unit and have set forth their experiences with the therapeutic modalities utilized in acute coronary care.[†] Information is also available dealing with the initial and continuing training of specialized nursing and medical personnel for the operation of coronary care facilities.[‡] In many instances treatment of the various arrhythmias and other complications of acute myocardial

---

[*]References: 2, 3, 5, 14–16, 37, 105, 106, 114, 195–197, 201–203, 206, 208, 210–215, 244.
[†]References: 2, 3, 5, 6, 14–16, 26, 37, 105, 106, 112, 140, 194–199, 201–205, 207, 209–215, 247–249, 254, 255, 265.
[‡]References: 2–5, 109–112, 114, 192, 193, 272.

infarction offers several options. In situations in which one type of treatment for a given situation has apparently been proved superior to other types of treatment, this will be noted as *treatment of choice*. Attempts have also been made to present the various *alternative methods* of therapy currently available.

There is a great deal of investigation to be done and many advances are yet to be made in the therapy of several aspects of acute myocardial infarction as carried out in the coronary care unit.

PART I

Acute Myocardial Infarction and Its Complications

CHAPTER 1

Functions of the Acute Coronary Care Unit

All complications of acute myocardial infarction occurring in the coronary care unit are related either to mechanical or electrical inefficiency or to failure of the heart in its ultimate function as a biologic pump. All therapeutic measures in the coronary care unit are ultimately planned for and directed toward the prevention or treatment of either mechanical or electrical inefficiency or failure of the heart-pump mechanism, whether that treatment be cardiopulmonary resuscitation or the administration of a laxative.

ESSENTIAL FUNCTIONS

1. Preventing Complications

The early detection and active prophylactic therapy of the known fatal and potentially fatal complications of acute myocardial infarction are the essential functions of the coronary care unit.

It has been estimated that coronary care units could save over 100,000 lives annually in the United States. This is a significant percentage of the Americans who die each year of myocardial infarction. This dramatic change in mortality due to myocardial infarction probably will not be achieved by more efficient resuscitation of the patient with cardiac arrest. Such change will be accomplished by *prevention* of these cardiac arrests. The prevention of cardiac arrests is the essential function of the coronary care unit and the function which could not be accomplished without close nurse monitoring of the electrocardiographic and other physiologic and psychologic parameters of each patient.

2. Electronic Monitoring

Electronic monitoring systems (ECG monitoring) initially provided the diagnostic modality which led to the establishment of intensive coronary care units.

The most valuable function of electronic monitoring systems is to provide the possibility of detecting early warning signs which forecast the possible occurrence of death-producing arrhythmias. Thereby we are offered the opportunity to treat the changed electrical status of the heart prophylactically with the hope of preventing a primary electrical cardiac death in the presence of an otherwise "good heart." The occurrence of electrical compromise of the heart beat is usually followed by some degree of secondary mechanical compromise. In the presence of primarily mechanical failure of the heart, electrical failure may be absent or may be a secondary or terminal event which is not reversible or treatable by available methods.

3. Clinical Investigation

An additional function of the coronary care unit is, of course, to study further and to define the disease process of acute myocardial infarction. It is hoped that continuing study will *provide further information* to anticipate complications more accurately and prevent death and disability from acute myocardial infarction in the future. These studies must be accomplished without causing harm, and with the hope of providing benefit, to the patient under investigation.

THERAPEUTIC MEASURES

Therapeutic measures are designed to aid in preventing the severe complications of acute myocardial infarction, thus better enabling the patient to survive the first very critical days of potential electrical and mechanical cardiac compromise which follow acute myocardial infarction. The first days are critical because of the potential dangers caused by heart muscle damage and necrosis, with resultant heart-pump and electrical mechanism alterations.

Therapeutic measures are aimed at minimizing the work requirements of the injured heart muscle and preventing disadvantageous stimulation of the patient and his heart which might result in the increased possibility of abnormal mechanical or electrical activity of the heart.

While general therapeutic measures are instituted, the electronic monitoring process has already been started in order to detect early warning signs of serious arrhythmias, so that early prophylactic therapy may be undertaken in the hope of preventing life-threatening arrhythmias.

CAUSES OF MECHANICAL OR ELECTRICAL FAILURE (IMMEDIATE LIFE-THREATENING COMPLICATIONS)

The types of mechanical or electrical heart-pump mechanism failure causing nearly all deaths in the hospital from acute myocardial infarction are:

MECHANICAL FAILURE CAUSES
1. Pulmonary edema
2. Congestive heart failure
3. Cardiogenic shock
4. Rupture of the myocardium
   a. Ventricle
   b. Intraventricular septum
   c. Papillary muscle

ELECTRICAL FAILURE CAUSES
Arrhythmias—all types
   a. Supraventricular tachyarrhythmias
   b. Ventricular ectopic arrhythmias
   c. Bradycardias and asystole

BOTH OR EITHER CAUSE
Thromboembolic phenomenon
   a. Cardiac origin
   b. Peripheral origin

DISCUSSION

Since the major risk of mortality from acute myocardial infarction occurs early in the infarction process, the benefit of a coronary care unit depends on early admission of patients with suspected myocardial infarction. This will necessarily lead to many false diagnoses. This is perfectly acceptable. Most coronary care units have up to a 50% misdiagnosis rate. Lower misdiagnosis rates probably mean that some patients with acute myocardial infarction are not being admitted to the coronary care unit at the time in their disease when they are most vulnerable to the life-threatening complications.

For those patients who are ultimately proved to have acute myocardial infarction, the length of time spent in the intensive coronary care unit will usually range from 3 to 7 days when the clinical course is uncomplicated, perhaps longer if the clinical course is complicated.

In caring for the patient with acute myocardial infarction we are concerned, in the acute coronary care unit, with a very short but important time span in the clinical spectrum of the patient's disease. We are also concerned with the period of time when the most serious complications may arise, even before an accurate diagnosis of acute myocardial infarction can be established clinically. Therefore it is wise to assume that all patients admitted for acute coronary care have had an actual acute myocardial infarction until proved otherwise.

CHAPTER 2

Physiology Related to Acute Coronary Care

Introduction

It is necessary to review some of the aspects of normal physiology in order to understand the pathologic processes and the effects of the various therapeutic measures on the cardiovascular system and autonomic nervous system in the presence of acute myocardial infarction.

The normal heart has four inherent properties: (1) excitability (irritability); (2) rhythmicity (automaticity); (3) conductivity; (4) contractility.

The heart operates as a twin pump mechanism. The right side of the heart pumps to the pulmonary circulation and the left side to the systemic circulation.

The rhythmic activity of the heart is normally maintained and regulated by a pacemaker located in the sinoatrial (SA) node.] SA

The normal physiologic functions of the heart are not merely the functions of the heart isolated from the remainder of the body but rather the functioning heart as it interacts with the effects of all the other organ systems.

For our purposes we will divide the *normal* physiologic functions of the heart into the following categories:
1. Initiation and conduction of the cardiac impulse.
2. Muscle contractility.
3. Autonomic nervous system.
4. Central nervous system control.

Fig. 1.—Normal conduction pathway.

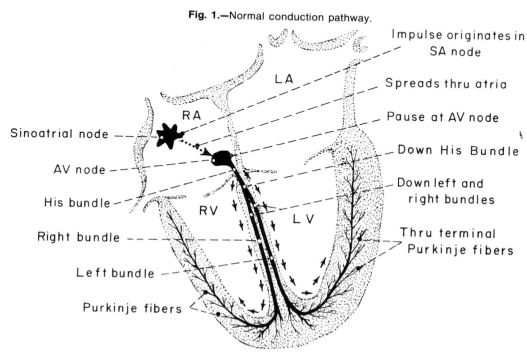

Sinoatrial node

AV node

His bundle

Right bundle

Left bundle

Purkinje fibers

LA

RA

RV   LV

Impulse originates in SA node

Spreads thru atria

Pause at AV node

Down His Bundle

Down left and right bundles

Thru terminal Purkinje fibers

Initiation and Conduction of the Cardiac Impulse*

SPECIALIZED CELLS

The conduction system of the heart is composed of *specialized* cells.
1. These specialized cells have properties different from those of the majority of myocardial cells, as follows:
   a. Ability to conduct impulses more rapidly than regular myocardial cells.
   b. Capacity to function as pacemakers which initiate the impulses that activate the heart muscle.
2. Regular, nonspecialized myocardial cells comprise the bulk of heart muscle.

CONDUCTION PATHWAY

In the normal heart the cardiac impulse travels by way of the following pathway (Fig. 1):
1. Impulse initiated in the SA node.
2. Spreads through the atrial muscles, which then contract.
   a. There are several identified special pathways through the atrial muscle by which the impulse may pass.
3. Undergoes a brief pause at the AV node.
4. Passes down the bundle of His.
5. Descends through the right and left bundle branches.
6. Reaches and spreads through the terminal Purkinje fibers, after which
7. The ventricle contracts.

ARTERIAL BLOOD SUPPLY TO SPECIALIZED CONDUCTION TISSUES

1. Anatomy of the arterial blood supply may be found in standard texts of anatomy and cardiology and other sources.[2,13,77]
2. Distribution.
   a. SA node: 50–60% from a branch of right coronary artery;
      40–50% from the left coronary artery.
   b. AV node: 90–92% by the right coronary artery;
      8–10% by a twig from circumflex branch, left coronary artery.

*References: 2, 5, 13, 71, 77.

   c. Bundle of His
      1) Left bundle branch–supplied by branches of both left and right coronary arteries.
      2) Right bundle branch–supplied by a branch of the anterior descending portion of the left coronary artery.

Normal Muscle Contracture†

BIOPHYSIOLOGY

1. Each cell contains mitochondria, sarcoplasm and fibrils.
2. Contractility of myocardial muscle cells is accomplished by their protein molecules.
3. These protein molecules respond to excitation and the cellular metabolic process by *releasing* metabolic energy in the form of *work* (i.e., myocardial contraction).

ENERGY-PRODUCING ENZYME MECHANISMS

1. Mitochondrial system.
   a. An enzyme oxidative phosphorylation system for oxidation of metabolites, for release of high-energy phosphate compounds (adenosine triphosphate; ATP).
   b. This system releases more energy for the same amount of metabolite than does the sarcoplasm system.
2. Sarcoplasm system. This system contains soluble enzymes involved in glycolysis (mostly anaerobic).

METABOLIC CYCLE	ENZYME INVOLVED	Measured to determine ACUTE MYOCARDIAL INFARCT
Glucose		
↓ ←− − − − 1. Lactic dehydrogenase − − − − − − − − − − −		(LDH)
↓ ←− − − − 2. Alpha-hydroxybutyrate dehydrogenase − − − −		(HBD)
Lactate + ATP → (high energy)		

3. Myokinase enzyme system.
   a. Cardiac muscle is rich in the following:
      1) Myoglobin.
      2) The enzymes of the tricarboxylic acid cycle (adenylic acid kinase).
      3) The electron transport system.
   b. Metabolic chemical reaction (highly reversible).

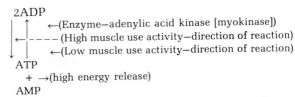

2ADP
←(Enzyme—adenylic acid kinase [myokinase])
− − − − (High muscle use activity—direction of reaction)
←(Low muscle use activity—direction of reaction)
ATP
  + →(high energy release)
AMP

†References: 8, 71, 77, 91, 251.

4. Creatine-creatine phosphate high energy system.

METABOLIC REACTION	ENZYME INVOLVED	Measured to determine ACUTE MYOCARDIAL INFARCT

Creatine phosphate + ADP
↓   ←‒‒‒‒‒‒‒‒‒(creatine phosphokinase)‒‒‒·‒‒(CPK)
Creatine + ATP→(high energy release)

MUSCLE CONTRACTION SYSTEM

1. The fibrils contain myosin and actin.
2. Actin and myosin are the protein substances which actually contract.
3. Myosin is an adenosine triphosphatase (ATPase) active protein (ATPase enzyme binds myosin and actin).
4. ATPase catalyzes hydrolysis of ATP, yielding energy.
5. During fibril contraction potassium ion leaves the myocardial cell.
6. During fibril relaxation potassium ion re-enters the myocardial cell.
7. Calcium has a positive inotropic effect on cardiac contractility.
8. Calcium affects cardiac depolarization by maintaining and regulating selective permeability of the myocardial cell membrane, particularly to sodium and potassium ions.[91]
9. Calcium probably affects myocardial cell membrane permeability by binding to the cell membrane in some manner.
10. Calcium is probably involved in all 3 of the major stages of myocardial contraction, namely
    a. Excitation (depolarization).
    b. Excitation–contraction coupling.
    c. Mechanical contraction.

11. Chemical reaction representing myocardial muscle contraction.

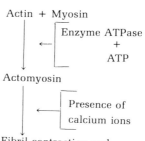

Actin + Myosin
↓   ← [Enzyme ATPase + ATP]
Actomyosin
↓   ← [Presence of calcium ions]
Fibril contraction and shortening (i.e., work from energy)

12. Pathologic physiology.
    a. Drugs which inhibit depolarization act by stabilizing myocardial cell membrane permeability, presumably by increasing calcium attachment to the cell membrane.
       1) Among drugs that inhibit depolarization are quinidine, procainamide and lidocaine.
    b. These drugs probably affect all 4 inherent properties of the heart.

SUMMARY OF BIOCHEMICAL PROCESSES OF MYOCARDIAL MUSCLE CONTRACTION

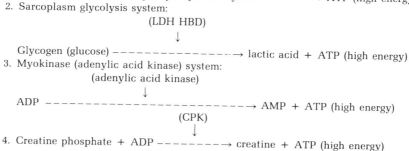

ENERGY PRODUCTION MECHANISM

1. Mitochondrial oxidative phosphorylation system ‒‒‒‒‒‒→ ATP (high energy)
2. Sarcoplasm glycolysis system:
    (LDH HBD)
    ↓
    Glycogen (glucose) ‒‒‒‒‒‒‒‒‒‒‒‒‒·‒→ lactic acid + ATP (high energy)
3. Myokinase (adenylic acid kinase) system:
    (adenylic acid kinase)
    ↓
    ADP ‒‒‒‒‒‒‒‒‒‒‒‒‒‒‒‒‒‒‒‒‒‒→ AMP + ATP (high energy)
    (CPK)
    ↓
4. Creatine phosphate + ADP ‒‒‒‒‒‒‒→ creatine + ATP (high energy)

MUSCLE CONTRACTION MECHANISM

calcium
Actin + myosin (ATPase) + ATP ‒‒‒‒‒‒‒‒→ Actomyosin contracted (work from energy)
ions

PATHOLOGIC CHANGE AND ENZYMATIC
DIAGNOSIS

In acute myocardial infarction the cardiac muscle cells of the affected area die (necrosis). When this occurs enzymes are released into the bloodstream from the necrotic muscle cells.

The schema at the bottom of page 9 reveals the normal site of biochemical activity of enzymes (CPK, LDH, HBD) in cardiac muscle metabolism. An additional enzyme (SGOT) is active in amino acid (protein) metabolism and is also released when myocardial cell death occurs.

Autonomic Nervous System[‡]

INTRODUCTION

The autonomic nervous system exerts great influence on the heart, blood vessels and lungs and therefore must be understood in order to gain an understanding of the physiology of the heart, the influence of acute myocardial infarction (AMI) on the heart, and the pharmacology of drugs affecting the heart in either normal or pathologic states.

DEFINITION AND DIVISIONS

The nervous system can be divided into 3 general systems. No one of these systems is entirely independent of the others. The systems are (1) central nervous system (CNS), (2) somatic nervous system and (3) autonomic nervous system.

1. **Definition.** The autonomic nervous system (also called visceral, vegetative and involuntary nervous system) consists of nervous tissue which supplies innervation to the heart, blood vessels, lungs, viscera, glands and smooth muscle. This system controls the so-called *automatic* functions of the body (Fig. 2).
2. **Divisions.** The autonomic nervous system consists of 2 divisions, the *parasympathetic* nervous system and the *sympathetic* nervous system.

‡References: 7, 14, 65, 71, 78, 81, 82, 92, 93, 126, 128, 129, 231.

The autonomic nervous system is separable anatomically, physiologically and pharmacologically into these 2 divisions—parasympathetic and sympathetic.[133] These systems generally oppose each other as physiologic antagonists,[7] thus maintaining the balanced physiologic status seen in normal cardiac function. If one system inhibits a certain function, the other system usually augments that function.

The parasympathetic division has few cardiovascular effects, with the effects of the vagus nerve being of chief importance. Stimulation of the vagus nerve slows the heart rate (negative chronotropic effect).

The sympathetic division plays a major role in regulation of blood pressure and blood flow by way of its action on vascular smooth muscle and its direct action on the heart.

The sympathetic division is further divided into 2 types of activity responses. These 2 types of responses are initiated and determined by activation of the respective receptor sites. The receptors are arbitrarily referred to as alpha and beta adrenergic receptors. They have not yet been defined by their physical, chemical staining or morphologic properties, but have been defined with respect to activity by extensive investigation.[7,93] (See Alpha and Beta Adrenergic Receptors, later in this section.)

AUTONOMIC NERVOUS SYSTEM ANATOMY

1. Afferent and Efferent Fibers and Impulses

Both the sympathetic and parasympathetic autonomic divisions have nerve fibers carrying nerve impulses *toward* and *away from* the central nervous system. The *afferent* nerve fibers carry the nerve impulses *to* the CNS and the *efferent* fibers carry the nerve impulses *from* the CNS.

The afferent fibers consist of strands of 1-cell length, and the efferent fibers consist of strands of 2-cell lengths, the 2 cells being arranged end-to-end and carrying the nerve impulse continuously over the length of the cells via synapse, without significant pause (Fig. 3).

Fig. 2.—Schematic representation of divisions of the autonomic nervous system.

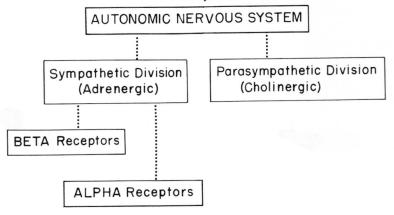

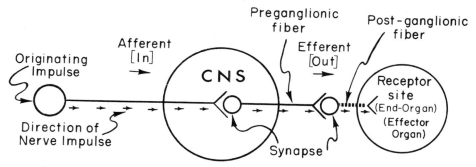

Fig. 3.—Schematic representation of the flow of a nerve impulse through afferent and efferent fibers and the involved synapses.

2. Afferent Fibers

The *afferent* fibers of the autonomic nervous system come from all parts of the body and are carried by the peripheral nerves and cranial nerves to the spinal cord and brain, respectively, making a variety of currently known and unknown connections before influencing the efferent impulses. The afferent fibers affecting the ultimate function of the *heart* originate predominantly from the following sites:

a. Vascular system (blood vessels) particularly the aortic arch and carotid sinus and bifurcation. Effects are from 2 types of receptors:
   1) Pressoreceptors (baroreceptors), representing the blood pressure effects at these sites.
   2) Chemoreceptors, affected by the blood pH, oxygen tension and carbon dioxide tension.
b. The heart itself, as influenced by the pressoreceptors in the ventricle and atrial walls.
c. The lungs, as influenced by the act of respiration and by the oxygen and carbon dioxide tensions present in the lungs.

The afferent fibers exert their effect predominantly on the centers located in the medulla (brain stem) of the central nervous system. (See Central Nervous System Control, later in this section.)

3. Efferent Fibers

a. The *efferent* fibers of the *parasympathetic* system affecting the *heart* originate in the brain stem and are carried to the heart via the vagus nerves. where they join with the second neuron of the 2-neuron efferent system. This second fiber group ends in direct action position to the heart muscle.
b. The *efferent* fibers of the *sympathetic* system affecting the *heart* originate in the upper thoracic segment of the spinal cord and are carried to the paravertebral ganglia as the preganglionic fibers. In the paravertebral ganglia they join with the second neuron of the efferent fiber system called the postganglionic fiber and are carried to the heart, where they end in direct action position to the heart muscle.

CHEMICAL BASIS FOR TRANSMISSION OF NERVE IMPULSES

The parasympathetic and sympathetic systems affect all 4 of the inherent properties of the heart (i.e., excitability, rhythmicity, conductivity and contractility). These effects are ultimately accomplished by the chemical-enzyme interactions that transmit the actual electrical nerve impulse. It is toward this chemical-enzyme molecular level that the effects of cardiovascular therapy are directed.

1. Parasympathetic Division

In the parasympathetic nervous system the chemically active molecule which mediates the nerve impulse at the heart is acetylcholine. Acetylcholine is destroyed by the enzyme cholinesterase. The chemically

Fig. 4.—Chemical mediation of a nerve impulse in the parasympathetic division of the autonomic nervous system.

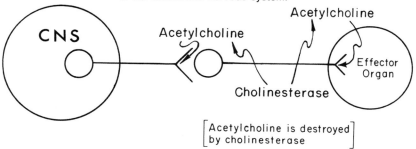

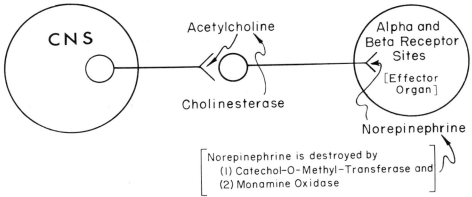

Fig. 5.—Chemical mediation of a nerve impulse in the sympathetic division of the autonomic nervous system.

active molecule at the end of the first neuron in the 2-neuron system is also acetylcholine. These relationships are schematically represented in Figure 4.

2. Sympathetic Division

It is generally accepted that the chemically active neurotransmitter molecule which mediates the sympathetic nerve impulse at the heart is norepinephrine.[7,133] This is the substance released by the arrival of a nerve impulse at the peripheral sympathetic receptor site. The enzymes which destroy norepinephrine are (1) catechol-O-methyl-transferase and (2) monoamine oxidase. However, these 2 enzymes do not destroy norepinephrine rapidly enough to account for its cessation of effect. The chemically active substance at the end of the first neuron in the 2-neuron system is acetylcholine, as in the parasympathetic system. Norepinephrine is a catecholamine. These relationships are schematically represented in Figure 5.

3. Somatic Muscle System

The neuromuscular transmission of nerve impulse for somatic (voluntary) muscle is entirely mediated by acetylcholine This is a reversible reaction and is schematically represented in Figure 6.

Fig. 6.—Chemical mediation of the neuromuscular transmission of nerve impulses for somatic (voluntary) muscle.

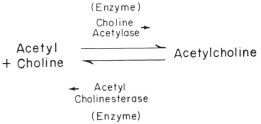

4. Cardiac Muscle

Both *cardiac* muscle and smooth muscle normally show *intrinsic* activity. It is theorized that this activity is regulated by acetylcholine which is synthesized and released by the muscle fibers themselves. This theory is based on the nature of the intrinsic muscle activity. Evidence for this theory is as follows:[71]

   a. This activity is both electrical and mechanical (see Normal Muscle Contracture).

   b. This activity is in contrast to other cholinergically innervated cells (i.e., autonomic neurons and skeletal muscle).

   c. This intrinsic activity is modified by nerve impulses but is *not* initiated by nerve impulses.

General Physiology of the Cardiac Autonomic Nervous System

   1. Parasympathetic (Vagal) Cardiac Stimulation[7,82,133,231]

     a. The vagus nerves represent the entire parasympathetic innervation of the heart.

     b. Vagal stimulation (parasympathetic cardiac stimulation)—effect on SA node:

       1) Produces bradycardia and other variable physiologic changes which are dependent on the strength of the stimulus.

       2) During vagal stimulation or acetylcholine application, single-cell microelectrode recordings in the SA node have shown decreased ability of spontaneous depolarization in pacemaker cells, thus causing bradycardia (inhibition of SA node).

     c. With vagal stimulation there are a decrease in atrial contractility, inhibition of atrial excitability and usually an increase in atrial conduction velocity.

     d. Vagal stimulation causes a decrease (inhibition) in conduction velocity in the AV node.

e. With vagal stimulation there is no sign of vagal influence on the His bundle, Purkinje system or ventricular cells as shown by microelectrode recordings.

f. With vagal stimulation the catecholamines released from the adrenal medulla are distributed diffusely to affect the sympathetic receptors and reinforce the action of the locally released neurotransmitter norepinephrine.

g. Summary—cardiac effect of parasympathetic stimulation:
   1) Vagal stimulation produces bradycardia (inhibition of SA node).
      a) May produce sinus arrest.
   2) There is decreased atrial contractility.
   3) There is increased atrial conduction velocity.
   4) There is decreased AV nodal conduction velocity (inhibition).
      a) May produce heart block.
   5) Vagal stimulation does *not* affect intraventricular condition.
   6) There is diffusely distributed catecholamine release from the adrenal medulla.

2. Sympathetic Cardiac Stimulation (Beta Stimulation)[7,82]

a. Sympathetic cardiac stimulation causes an increase in the efficiency of work performed by the heart in both atria and ventricles via the following mechanisms.
   1) Decrease in left ventricular systolic and diastolic dimensions (increased inotropy).
   2) Abrupt increase in left ventricular systolic pressure with no increase in left ventricular diastolic pressure.
   3) Abrupt tachycardia.
   4) Increase in left ventricular stroke work and output per minute (i.e., contractility).
   5) More vigorous atrial contractions.
   6) Increase in oxygen demand of the heart.
b. Sympathetic cardiac stimulation produces coronary vasodilation.
c. Sympathetic cardiac stimulation shortens the atrial-to-His bundle conduction interval (increase atrial conduction velocity).
d. Sympathetic cardiac stimulation has minimal effects on the AV node, His bundle, Purkinje and intraventricular conduction time.
e. Summary—Effect of Cardiac Sympathetic Stimulation:
   1) Increases work efficiency of the heart.
   2) Dilates the coronary arteries.
   3) Shortens the SA-to-AV conduction time (i.e., increases atrial conduction velocity, shortens PR ECG interval).

4) Minimally affects AV node or intraventricular conduction.
5) Increases oxygen demand.

Alpha and Beta Adrenergic Receptors[§]

1. Definition

The sympathetic nervous system has been further divided into 2 distinctive types of receptors at the effector organ site. The 2 types of receptors have been arbitrarily called alpha and beta adrenergic receptors, served by like alpha and beta adrenergic fibers. These receptors are affected (blocked or stimulated) by various drugs and have opposite functions within the sympathetic nervous system when individually stimulated. The concept of alpha and beta adrenergic receptors was clearly defined by Ahlquist[129] in 1948 after being investigated for a number of years.

In normal and pathologic states the alpha and beta adrenergic receptors are stimulated endogenously by norepinephrine as the sympathetic neurohumoral transmitter available at the receptor sites and by epinephrine, which is released from the medulla of the adrenal gland when sympathetic nervous system stimulation occurs. Effects of these 2 naturally occurring catecholamines are simulated to varying degrees by all sympathomimetic amines utilized in therapy of cardiovascular conditions. Alpha and beta receptors may be individually stimulated or blocked by various chemicals utilized in drug therapy.

2. Hypothesis of Chemical Mechanism for Alpha and Beta Receptor Activity

a. Sympathomimetic amine (see prototype formula, Fig. 7) enters the effector cell activating the specific alpha or beta receptors.
b. The membrane enzyme adenyl cyclase catalyzes the reaction of ATP to 3′, 5′ cyclic AMP.[14]
   1) The 3′, 5′ cyclic AMP activates several enzymes as follows:
      a) Phosphorylase.
      b) Phosphofructokinase.
      c) Lipase.
c. Alpha or beta adrenergic stimulation occurs.

3. Physiologic Effects of Alpha and Beta Stimulation

Understanding of the effects of general sympathetic stimulation and of alpha and beta adrenergic stimulation is necessary to the understanding of the pharmacophysiologic action of many drugs utilized for therapy in acute coronary care. The comprehension of these

§References: 7, 14, 92, 93, 128, 129.

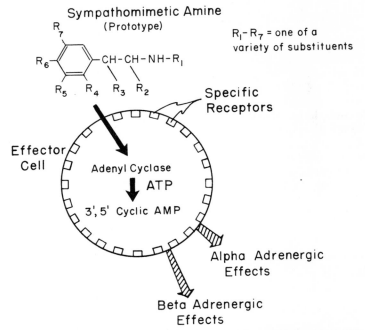

Fig. 7.—Schema of the chemical mechanism of alpha and beta adrenergic receptor stimulation.

effects is particularly necessary to the understanding of the pathologic physiology and treatment of shock. Some specifics in this regard follow:

    a. Sympathomimetic amines: definition (see Glossary).

    b. Generally, stimulation of *alpha* adrenergic receptors has sympathetic *excitatory* effects.

    c. Generally, stimulation of *beta* adrenergic receptors has sympathetic *inhibitory* effects.

    d. Exceptions to the above effects of stimulation are as follows:[7,128]

       1) *Beta receptors* to the *heart* manifest entirely *excitatory* effects when stimulated by sympathomimetic amines.

TABLE 1.—EFFECTS OF ALPHA AND BETA ADRENERGIC STIMULATION

EFFECTOR ORGAN	RECEPTOR TYPE	STIMULATION RESPONSE
Heart		
SA node	Beta	Increased heart rate (chronotropic effect)
AV node	Beta	a) Increased conduction velocity b) Decreased refractory period
Atria	Beta	Increased contraction strength (inotropic effect)
Ventricles	Beta	Increased contraction strength (inotropic effect)
Blood vessels*		
Coronary	Alpha and beta	Dilatation
Cerebral	Alpha	Constriction (very slight)
Pulmonary	Alpha	Constriction
Skin and mucosal	Alpha	Constriction
Renal†	Alpha	Constriction
Abdominal viscera†	Alpha	Constriction
Skeletal muscle†,‡	Beta	Dilatation
Lung		
Bronchial muscle	Beta	Relaxation

    *The effect on the blood vessels is through the sympathetic nervous system effect on the *smooth muscle* of blood vessels.

    †Represents the neurophysiologic effects when the neurotransmitters are present in concentrations *over* the usual physiologic range. This does not apply to the liver, in the case of "abdominal viscera."

    ‡Skeletal muscle vasculature represents a great deal of the total arterial vascular network, thus the *over-all* effect of beta adrenergic stimulation is vasodilatation.

2) Inhibitory effects of sympathomimetic amines on the gut are mediated by both alpha and beta receptors.

e. Complete tables are available showing the responses to alpha and beta stimulation of all organs of the body.[7,92,128] However, for our purposes in dealing with the patient requiring acute coronary care, we are concerned with the responses of the heart, blood vessels and lungs, along with the therapeutic modalities for altering these responses.

f. Table 1 shows the effects of alpha and beta adrenergic stimulation on the important effector organs related to acute coronary care. Blockade would, of course, produce the opposite effects.[7,14,92,128]

CATECHOLAMINES

1. The catecholamines[7,14,65,78,81] norepinephrine, epinephrine and isoproterenol are phenylethanolamines containing 2 hydroxyl groups on the benzene ring (Fig. 8).
   a. Chemical structures (Fig. 8).
      1) Catechol is the basic structural unit.
      2) Norepinephrine is phenylethanolamine with 2 hydroxyl groups on the benzene ring.
      3) Epinephrine has an additional methyl group attached to the amine.
      4) Isoproterenol has an isopropyl radical attached to the amine (synthetic).
   b. Norepinephrine and epinephrine occur naturally in man.
      1) Norepinephrine is synthesized in the cells of the sympathetic nervous system and adrenal medulla.
      2) Epinephrine is released from the adrenal medulla as part of adrenergic sympathetic control.
   c. The catecholamines mediate their effect through the alpha and beta adrenergic receptors of the sympathetic nervous system.
      1) Norepinephrine and epinephrine mediate via both alpha and beta receptors.
         a) Norepinephrine mediates greater alpha activity.
         b) Epinephrine mediates greater beta activity.
      2) Isoproterenol mediates via beta receptors only.

d. The steps in the enzymatic synthesis of norepinephrine and epinephrine are shown in Figure 9.

2. Sympathomimetic Amines

Beta-phenylethylamine can be viewed as the parent compound of the sympathomimetic amines.[7]

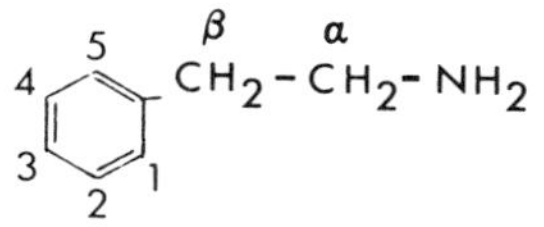

Beta-phenylethylamine

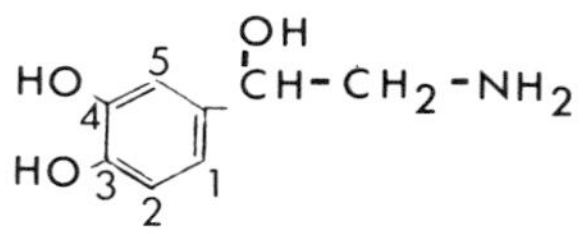

Catecholamine (norepinephrine)

a. With an OH group on positions 3 and 4 of the benzene ring, the compound becomes a catecholamine.

b. Sympathomimetic amines include by common usage all of the compounds referred to as vasoconstrictor amines, vasopressor amines and catecholamines.

c. Vasoconstrictor amines are those sympathomimetic amines which stimulate alpha receptors only, to affect only the blood vessels, and have no inotropic or chronotropic properties. However, by common usage this group has come to mean all sympathomimetic amines.

d. Vasopressor amines strictly speaking should be used as a term synonymous with vasoconstrictor amines. However, by common usage the term is usually applied to all sympathomimetic amines which produce vasoconstriction as part of their pharmacologic effect, regardless of other activities of the drug, and which are used in the treatment of shock. This includes vasoconstrictor amines and catecholamines.

3. Physiology of Catecholamines

a. Norepinephrine, metaraminol and isoproterenol are the most commonly used drugs in the treatment of cardiogenic shock. (Metaraminol is not a catecholamine.)
   1) It should be noted that the mechanism of action of metaraminol is via displacement of norepinephrine from its endogenous sites,[126] and in effect norepinephrine is the active

Fig. 8.—Chemical structures of catecholamines.

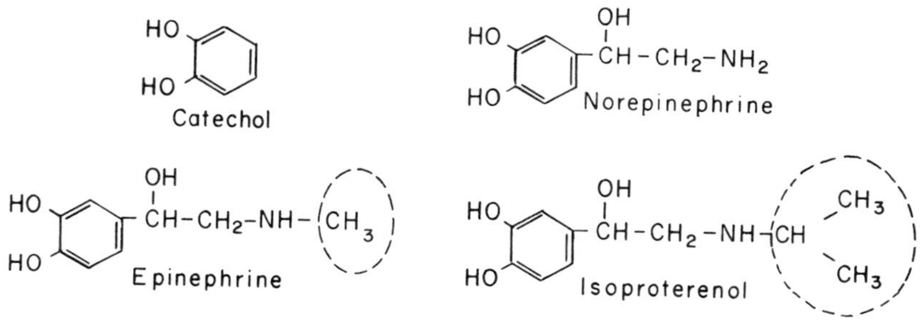

Catechol

Norepinephrine

Epinephrine

Isoproterenol

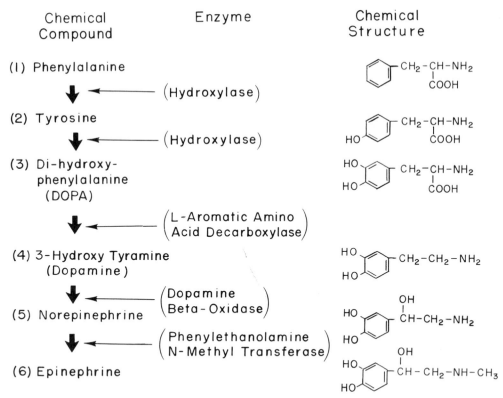

Fig. 9.—Steps in the enzymatic synthesis of norepinephrine and epinephrine.

chemical stimulator of the sympathetic nervous system in this particular type of therapy. Metaraminol is a norepinephrine-liberating (releasing) agent.

   b. Catecholamines induce variable metabolic and physiologic effects in the different organs. The nature and strength of these effects are dependent on the particular catecholamine and the organ system involved and primarily on whether alpha or beta receptor effects predominate.[7,81] Following is a comparison of the cardiovascular effects of the infusion of the catecholamines in the intact animal.

     1) *Norepinephrine.*
       a) Raises blood pressure.
       b) Slows heart rate–via carotid sinus reflex of blood pressure increase.
       c) Increases systemic vascular resistance.
       d) Increases cardiac output.

     2) *Epinephrine and Isoproterenol.*
       a) Blood pressure may increase, decrease or remain unchanged.
       b) Heart rate increases.
       c) Systemic vascular resistance may be unchanged or lowered.
       d) Cardiac output is increased.

Central Nervous System Control

INTRODUCTION

The central nervous system control of the heart is accomplished by way of the autonomic nervous system, which transports the stimulus originated in the central nervous system to the heart, blood vessels and lungs.

All portions of the brain seem to have some effect on the autonomic nervous system,[190] either directly or through the complex interaction of one area of the brain with another. These varied effects of separate areas of the brain are difficult or impossible to study in their entirety at present because of the complex nature of the central nervous system and because of its action as a whole and integrated organ system.

For our purposes we will consider the 3 major areas of central nervous system influence on the heart. These are the cerebral medulla, the hypothalamus and higher cerebral centers. Stimuli originating in the central nervous system ultimately act through the fibers of the autonomic nervous system to produce their effects.

CEREBRAL MEDULLA

The primary central nervous system control centers for autonomic activity of the heart, blood vessels and lungs are in the cerebral medulla (brain stem) of the brain.

Spontaneous activity of sympathetic fibers appears to reside in the cerebral medulla. Even after elimination of all afferent nerve pathways to this area a continuous neuronal discharge activity persists, in the presence of a normal chemical environment.[84]

The regular autonomic activity mediated by the cerebral medulla is controlled by a complex physiologic interaction of collections of nervous tissue centers located in the cerebral medulla and named:
1. The sympathetic cardiac accelerator center.
2. The parasympathetic cardiac inhibitory center.
3. The sympathetic vasoconstrictor center.

The afferent and efferent impulses related to these cerebral medullary centers exert their effect on heart rate, peripheral vasoconstriction and peripheral vasodilatation. These afferent and efferent impulses effected by the cerebral medullary centers are in equilibrium with and therefore influenced by changes in physiologic functions of the following:
1. Blood pH.
2. Blood Po_2.
3. Blood Pco_2.
4. Arterial pressure in the aortic arch and carotid sinus (carotid sinus reflex).
5. Venous pressure in the pulmonary veins, vena cava and right atrium (Bainbridge reflex).
6. Inspiratory and expiratory phases of respiration (Hering-Breuer reflex).
7. Probably by pressor–receptor fibers in the walls of the ventricles.

Hypothalamus

Electrical stimulation of various portions of the hypothalamus in experimental animals has presented a variety of cardiovascular and ECG activity, much too complex to consider in great detail here.

Some of the difficulties in appreciating the complexities of experimental hypothalamic stimulation may be seen from the fact that stimulation of various areas of the hypothalamus has produced the following results:[84]
1. Anterior hypothalamic stimulation has caused
   a. Bradycardia.
   b. Hypertension.
   c. ECG—ST elevation and T-wave inversion.
2. Lateral hypothalamic stimulation has caused
   a. Hypertension.
   b. AV dissociation.
   c. VPCs.
3. Posterolateral stimulation has caused
   a. Hypertension.
   b. AV nodal rhythm.
   c. Aberrant intraventricular conduction.
   d. VPCs.
Multiple experimental hypothalamic stimulation studies and ECG records taken during stimulation have

placed emphasis on the *intermingling* of vasopressor and vasodepressor areas of extremely small size in the hypothalamus and the *multiplicity* of cardiac responses obtained.[84] Tachycardia, bradycardia, ventricular tachycardia, multifocal VPCs, AV dissociation, tall T-waves, T-wave inversion, ST elevation and U-waves have all been seen.[115]

Experimental hypothalamic stimulation at various sites in the cat with study of the adrenal medullary secretion of epinephrine and norepinephrine has shown that some areas when stimulated provoke comparatively huge quantities of one or the other of these chemical mediators with a wide variation in the ratio of the epinephrine and norepinephrine.[116]

The fact that such a variety of cardiovascular and ECG activity occurs with microelectrode stimulation indicates that the hypothalamus is extremely important and influential on the heart and vascular system, though the exact nature of all these influences has not been well defined.

Higher Cerebral Centers

It is sufficient to state that many pathways from the higher cerebral centers which effect the cardiac and vascular responses have been demonstrated to relay their peripheral effects via both the hypothalamus and the cerebral medulla.[84] There are undoubtedly many pathways effecting cardiac and vascular responses which are unknown or ill defined at the present time.

A large variety of neurologic diseases has been incriminated as causing ECG abnormalities, particularly arrhythmias. These neurologic diseases might be considered the clinical counterparts of experimental neurogenic cardiac stimulation described above.[85] It must be concluded that neural influences may overtax the heart, particularly the acutely ill heart.

In an excellent, general review of the central autonomic influences[190] it is pointed out that the theory that the autonomic nervous system is an altogether automatic regulatory device unrelated to the integrative functions of the cerebral hemispheres is incorrect. The autonomic nervous system *is* affected by the integrative mechanisms of the higher centers of the brain, and the regulation of the autonomic nervous system *is not* automatic, but conversely is markedly influenced by a number of nonautomatic factors.

It appears that the regulatory activity of higher centers on the autonomic nervous system is manifest not by simple antagonism of the sympathetic and parasympathetic discharges but by coordinated patterning of impulses in both components of the autonomic nervous system. In fact, selective simultaneous activation of both cholinergic and adrenergic elements may frequently occur.[190]

It appears there may be an inhibitory restraint mediated by the higher central nervous system centers on the autonomic nervous system.

PATHOLOGIC PHYSIOLOGY

Stressful life experiences may impair the usual restraining influences of the higher centers on the autonomic nervous system, causing the autonomic nervous system to become hyperirritable.[190] In this regard, observations in a coronary care unit have shown a correlation of occurrence of arrhythmias with emotionally stressful events, such as conflicts with a wife during visiting hours or anxiety following emergency resuscitation of a neighbor.[190]

Anxiety if expressed via the autonomic nervous system through the cardiovascular system may start in the hypothalamus or higher cerebral centers.[77] The effects of anxiety on the cardiovascular system have been studied and it has been found that anxiety may produce increases in cardiac output, heart rate, oxygen consumption and peripheral resistance[59] as well as ECG changes.[120] These changes appear to be similar to those produced by small doses of epinephrine in some patients.

CHAPTER 3

Pathologic Physiology of Acute Myocardial Infarction

Introduction

The study of the pathologic physiology of acute myocardial infarction is the study of the effects of obstruction (or occlusion) of some portion of the coronary circulation. Since these effects in man can only be studied indirectly, investigative work in this field has proceeded on laboratory animals, particularly mammals. With the advent of continuous electrocardiographic monitoring of patients with acute myocardial infarction and the development of instrumentation for sophisticated study of the pathologic process of acute myocardial infarction in man, many of the observations made in laboratory animals have had clinical correlation and verification. A few of the study results in laboratory animals have been refuted by study in man.

In studying the pathologic physiology of acute myocardial infarction in man it has been morally necessary for the various investigators to hope to provide benefit to the patients who are being studied at the time they are studied, or at least to cause no harm. As a result, studies are limited in scope and the pathologic process occurring in a given patient is altered for the *benefit* of that patient, when this can be accomplished with current modalities of therapy.

Many of the results described in this section are derived from animal studies. This will not be specifically noted on each occasion unless it is deemed pertinent.

MECHANICAL DERANGEMENTS OF THE
MYOCARDIUM

After ligation of a coronary artery or its branch, the affected portion of myocardium undergoes significant changes in just 15–20 minutes. If the artery remains ligated for a longer time, the changes are irreversible. [12,71] The changes in mechanical function are as follows:
1. The affected myocardium appears cyanotic.
2. There is a failure of effective contractility, which adversely affects the heart's ability to perform work.
3. The ischemic and anoxic myocardium then ceases to participate in contraction.

a. It appears likely that one of the early effects of myocardial ischemia is failure of the excitation-contraction coupling mechanism. [12]
  1) This is the mechanism linking excitation at the cell surface to the contractile response of the myofilaments.
  2) The mechanism responsible for interruption in the link coupling excitation and contraction in the muscle is not known.
4. Following this, the affected portion of myocardium bulges paradoxically outward during systolic contraction. This further decreases the efficiency of the heart as a pump, dissipating energy into the affected area.
5. It may be tentatively concluded that hypotension (as manifest by cardiogenic shock) and heart failure (as manifest by pulmonary edema and congestive heart failure) reflect the effects of impaired myocardial performance.
6. Experimental coronary arteriography studies suggest that vasoconstriction occurs in both the occluded and nonoccluded coronary arteries. [77] This process contributes to further ischemia and less effective myocardial contraction.

METABOLIC DERANGEMENTS OF THE
MYOCARDIUM

1. *Aerobic Metabolism*

  a. The heart must normally provide its contractile apparatus with a constant supply of high-energy phosphate (see Normal Muscle Contracture in Chapter 2).
  b. These high-energy phosphates are produced primarily by effective oxidative pathways under aerobic metabolic conditions, and these aerobic pathways are dependent on a continuous delivery of oxygen.
  c. The continuous supply of oxygen must be delivered via the coronary circulation.

    1) With coronary occlusion this delivery system is shut off to a portion of the myocardium.

  d. There is no storage of oxygen in the myoglobin of heart muscle.

  e. Failure of the heart muscle to receive oxygen will thus bring the major energy-yielding reactions of myocardial metabolism to a halt in the affected area.

2. *Anaerobic Metabolism*

  a. Under conditions of acute myocardial infarction, there is activation of anaerobic metabolism.

  b. The ability of anaerobic metabolism to produce high-energy phosphate is relatively poor compared to aerobic metabolism.

  c. Numerous metabolic changes occur with the activation of the anaerobic mechanism.[12] These changes are as follows:

    1) There is increased activity of certain enzyme systems due to shift to anaerobic pathways of adenosine triphosphate (ATP) production. These enzyme systems are:
      a) Phosphofructokinase.
      b) Phosphorylase.
      c) Hexokinase.

    2) The phosphofructokinase enzyme system is stimulated by increases of inorganic phosphate and adenosine 5-monophosphate (AMP) occurring with anaerobiosis.

    3) Anoxic activation of the phosphorylase enzyme system causes glycogenolysis and a rapid reduction of cardiac muscle glycogen content.

    4) Anoxia is known to increase the myocardial uptake of glucose, thus providing additional substrate for anaerobic glycolysis. This activity reflects an increase in the hexokinase enzyme system.

    5) Lactate normally is consumed by the myocardium, but with anoxia and anaerobiosis there is a net increased production of lactate.

Fig. 10.—Schematic representation of the pathologic physiology of heart muscle contraction occurring with acute myocardial infarction.

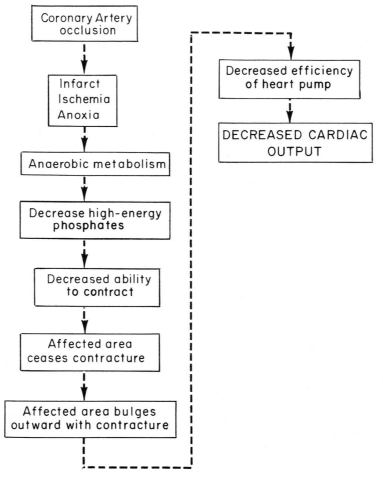

CONTRACTILITY DERANGEMENTS OF THE MYOCARDIUM

1. Biochemical Energy of Contraction[12]

a. From a biochemical viewpoint the heart is provided with a number of mechanisms by which the rate of ATP production can be increased following interruption of coronary arterial blood flow.

b. From a functional viewpoint, however, anaerobic energy production is inadequate for generation of useful cardiac work by *ischemic* heart muscle

c. The ultimate cause of impaired contractility of the ischemic heart is undoubtedly the decreased rate of high-energy phosphate production.

2. Pathologic Physiology of Contraction

A schematic representation of the pathologic physiology of heart muscle contraction occurring with acute myocardial infarction is seen in Figure 10.

3. Hemodynamic Changes and the Myocardial Contractile Defect

a. There is some degree of contractile defect of myocardial muscle in every instance of acute myocardial infarction. This contractile derangement is clinically notable in some patients; in other patients it is not clinically evident.

b. In most seriously ill patients with acute myocardial infarction the usual circulation (hemodynamic) abnormality is low cardiac output with increased peripheral vascular resistance.
   1) These hemodynamic changes may be associated with some degree of cardiogenic shock or pulmonary edema.
      a) In cardiogenic shock the systemic vascular resistance is often normal while the cardiac output is low.

c. Although myocardial contractility clearly plays an important role in the pathogenesis of abnormal states (complications) following acute myocardial infarction,[12] the results of studies reveal that the hemodynamic state following interruption of coronary arterial flow can be influenced to an important extent by factors *not* related to the myocardial contractile defect.[66] No completely consistent pattern of low cardiac output, high cardiac output or changes in peripheral resistance has been found to fit the various clinical situations in man.

d. The hemodynamic effects are probably predominantly related to the major complications which arise; however, major complications cannot as yet be forecast by measurable hemodynamic changes that follow acute myocardial infarction (cannot be predicted from hemodynamic studies in an individual patient).

CATECHOLAMINES AND ACUTE MYOCARDIAL INFARCTION

Increases in the urinary excretion of catecholamines (norepinephrine and epinephrine) in man during the acute phases of acute myocardial infarction have been demonstrated.[65,130] Animal experiments have also been carried out, and generally these have shown some increase in the circulating levels of catecholamines.[28,182] It is generally felt that there is some importance to the increase of catecholamines in the body following acute myocardial infarction, but the exact significance of this increase and the extent of its effect on the occurrence of complications (particularly arrhythmias) are not clear. It is generally found that the catecholamine increase is smallest in uncomplicated cases of acute myocardial infarction, and the greater increases almost always occur in the presence of complications, such as cardiogenic shock, pulmonary edema and arrhythmias.[252] The exact circumstances in which either norepinephrine or epinephrine individually may specifically increase is not well defined, but it is thought that an increase in epinephrine is more apt to be correlated with occurrence of an arrhythmia and an increase in norepinephrine with shock or pulmonary edema.[177] Additional investigation will be necessary to elucidate these relationships.

BLOOD OXYGEN TENSION AFTER ACUTE MYOCARDIAL INFARCTION[229]

1. Blood-tissue oxygen tension gradients are decreased in acute myocardial infarction. This decrease occurs in essentially all patients with acute myocardial infarction, particularly those with left ventricular failure,[246] and is brought about by the following:
   a. Disturbance of pulmonary function.
   b. Diminished tissue perfusion via decreased myocardial contractility.

2. Pulmonary function tends to deteriorate in the first 3 days after admission of patients with acute myocardial infarction. It is thought that there is lowered pulmonary diffusing capacity.[246]

3. It is probable that a disturbance of ventilation-perfusion is responsible for the altered lung function.
   a. There is an abnormally large venous admixture effect in patients after acute myocardial infarction. This occurs via one of the following:
      1) Blood being shunted past functioning lung tissues, or
      2) The admixture of blood from areas of low ventilation-perfusion ratios.

4. Initial pulmonary disturbance is more serious in the presence of pulmonary edema.

a. Lung function in these patients with pulmonary edema may show improvement over several weeks after pulmonary edema has resolved radiographically.
b. The acute changes are influenced by diuretic and other supportive therapy.
c. Pulmonary function often deteriorates in the first few days, at a time when pulmonary congestion is resolving.

OTHER SOURCES OF PATHOLOGIC PHYSIOLOGY INFORMATION

Discussions of the pathologic physiology occurring with the immediate life-threatening complications of cardiogenic shock, pulmonary edema and arrhythmias will be found in the part of this manual dealing with complications. A review of the pathologic physiology of cardiogenic shock will be particularly helpful in understanding the general pathophysiologic changes occurring with acute myocardial infarction.

CHAPTER 4

Arrhythmias

Introduction

Arrhythmias are the most common of the life-threatening or potentially life-threatening complications of acute myocardial infarction. Some type of arrhythmic disturbance occurs in as high as 90–95% of patients monitored in the coronary care unit.[32,242] Arrhythmias as a group have been responsible for a larger number of in-hospital deaths than any of the other complications of acute myocardial infarction. The procedure of continuous ECG monitoring in the acute coronary care unit has provided more information with regard to treatment of arrhythmias than for any of the other complications of acute myocardial infarction. Electrocardiographic monitoring in the coronary care unit has also permitted early recognition and active treatment of serious arrhythmias, or prophylactic treatment of minor arrhythmias that are known to lead to potentially major, life-threatenting arrhythmias. It is in the area of *preventing* deaths caused by arrhythmias, with the salvage of more patients with otherwise good hearts, that the most important benefits of the coronary care unit have been realized. The hope for a decrease in mortality rate or in complications other than arrhythmias is concerned at the present only with earlier detection by virtue of closer nursing observation. The advent of the coronary care unit has not as yet significantly changed the mortality rate associated with other complications of acute myocardial infarction.

The methods of managing arrhythmias complicating acute myocardial infarction are similar to those used in the patient without infarction. The plan of action for treatment and the speed with which action must be taken are modified because of the ventricular insult associated with the acute myocardial infarction. Because of this ventricular insult (myocardial damage) and the susceptibility to cardiac arrhythmias and arrest arising out of disturbances of rhythm that would be of little or no importance in the healthy heart, all arrhythmias take on much greater significance and require greater urgency of treatment.[162] Examples may be seen in ven-

tricular extrasystoles and various AV blocks, which can lead to more serious arrhythmias.

Pathologic Physiology

In general, the cardiovascular hemodynamic effects of arrhythmias are as follows:

1. The *ventricular response rate* of an arrhythmia, regardless of the type, can be of great importance at either extreme of heart rate.

2. With the advent of continuous ECG monitoring of patients with acute myocardial infarction, new concepts of the frequency of occurrence of arrhythmias, as well as of the pathologic steps in the development of serious arrhythmias, have been discovered.

   By the procedure of continuous ECG monitoring, it has been found that in 90-95% of the patients with acute myocardial infarction some type and severity of arrhythmias develop.[26,32] The prognosis depends on the functional severity of the arrhythmia, and the propensity of the arrhythmia to lead to more serious arrhythmias. Various studies have demonstrated that, during the time of observation in the coronary care unit, a great number ot the patients with acute myocardial infarction have at least one incident of a serious primary arrhythmia, capable of causing significant deterioration in the hemodynamic state.

3. The decrease in mortality of patients managed in the coronary care unit has been primarily the result of prevention of the ectopic ventricular arrhythmias (premature ventricular contractions, ventricular tachycardia, ventricular fibrillation, and idioventricular rhythm associated with complete AV block) and thus of the cardiac arrest which frequently ensues.[26,105,106]

   Unfortunately, antiarrhythmic technics have not as yet significantly decreased the mortality in patients with intractable heart failure or cardiogenic shock following acute myocardial infarction.

4. The relationship of atrial systole to ventricular sys-

TABLE 2.—CLASSIFICATION OF ARRHYTHMIAS IN ACUTE MYOCARDIAL INFARCTION

Site of Origin	Disturbance in Rate and Conduction			Prognosis in AMI			Groups for Considering Therapy			
	Cardiac Impulse Formation	Ectopic	Cardiac Impulse Conduction	Minor	Major	Death-Producing Arrhythmia	Supra-ventricular	Ectopic Ventricular	Brady-arrhythmias	Requires No Therapy for Arrhythmia
Sinoatrial (SA) node										
Sinus arrhythmia				X						X
Sinus bradycardia	X				X				X	
Sinus tachycardia	X			X					X	
Sinus arrest	X				X				X	
SA block			X		X				X	
Atria										
PACs (less than 6/min.)	X	X		X			X			X
PACs (more than 6/min.)	X	X			X		X			
Atrial tachycardia	X	X			X		X			
Atrial tachycardia with block	X	X	X		X		X			
Atrial flutter	X	X	X		X		X			
Atrial fibrillation	X	X	X		X		X		X	
Atrial standstill	X								X	
Wandering pacemaker	X		X						X	
Intra-atrial block			X	X						X
Atrioventricular (AV) node										
PNCs (less than 6/min.)	X	X		X			X			X
PNCs (more than 6/min.)	X	X			X		X			
Nodal tachycardia	X	X			X		X			
Nodal tachycardia with retrograde block (AV dissociation)	X	X	X		X		X			
Delayed AV conduction (1st-degree heart block)			X	X						X
2d-degree AV heart block (2:1 or 3:1 block)			X		X				X	
Complete AV heart block (3d-degree block with nodal rhythm)	X		X		X				X	
Ventricles										
Idioventricular rhythm with 3d-degree block	X		X		X			X	X	
Infrequent PVCs in 1st 24 hr.	X	X			X			X	X	
PVCs (less than 6/min.) (after 24 hours)	X	X		X				X		X
PVCs (more than 6/min.)	X	X			X			X		
PVC salvos or multifocal	X	X			X			X		X
Bundle branch block	X		X		X					X
Ventricular tachycardia	X	X			X	X		X		
Ventricular fibrillation/flutter	X	X			X	X		X		
Ventricular standstill (asystole)	X		X							
a. Primary asystole			X		X	X				
b. Secondary asystole			X		X	X				

NOTE: PAC = premature atrial contractions; PNC = premature nodal contractions; PVC = premature ventricular contractions.

tole determines whether or not normal atrial transport function will be present and determines the efficiency of AV valve closure.

5. Efficiency of cardiac pumping would not be possible without coordinated contraction of the muscle mass which makes up the ventricular cylinder. Control of the regularity, rate and effectiveness of contraction depends largely on electrophysiologic mechanisms, including:
    a. Site of impulse formation.
    b. Regularity of electrical impulses.
    c. Relative synchrony of impulse conduction.[11]
        1) The site of origin and type of conduction of the pacing stimulus are important determinants of the effectiveness of ventricular systole and AV valve competency.
6. The pathologic condition of the heart as a pump determines how effectively and how long the adverse effects of arrhythmias may be tolerated.
7. The integrity of the vasomotor control mechanism serves as a final site of adjustment for maintaining adequate perfusion of the vital centers of the total patient. (See Autonomic Nervous System in Chapter 2; Chapter 5.)
8. Associated diseases determine how well a compromised circulation may be tolerated.
9. The total hemodynamic effect of the arrhythmia depends on the summation of effects of numerous changes of varying importance, and the effects of these changes on a given individual's pre-existing and present cardiovascular status.
10. Additional effects of arrhythmias on the hemodynamic function of the heart may be found under discussions of specific arrhythmias.

Classification of Arrhythmias

When one begins to study arrhythmias, it becomes rapidly apparent that many different methods of classification of arrhythmias, particularly in acute myocardial infarction, are used by various authors and investigators. In an attempt to clarify to some extent the classification and mechanisms of arrhythmias in acute myocardial infarction, these various methods of classification are presented in tabular form, as related to each of the arrhythmias (Table 2). Discussion of the arrhythmias will then follow, with division into groups for purposes of active treatment.

CRITERIA FOR CLASSIFICATION

For our purposes in considering therapy of the arrhythmias, it is probably best to view each arrhythmia from all points of classification. Arrhythmias are shown in Table 2 classified according to 4 different methods.[5,26,33,71,77]

1. *According to site of origin of arrhythmia:*
    a. Sinoatrial (SA) node.
    b. Atrial
    c. Atrioventricular (AV) node.
    d. Ventricle.
2. *Disturbance in cardiac rate and conduction, divided into:*
    a. Disturbances in cardiac impulse formation.
        1) Sinoatrial rhythms.
        2) Ectopic rhythms.
    b. Disturbances in cardiac impulse conduction.
3. *According to prognosis (specific for acute myocardial infarction):*
    a. Minor arrhythmia.
    b. Major arrhythmia.
    c. Death-producing arrhythmia.
4. *According to groups for consideration of therapy:*
    a. Supraventricular tachyarrhythmias.
        1) Paroxysmal atrial tachycardia.
        2) Auricular flutter or fibrillation.
        3) Nodal tachycardia.
    b. Ectopic ventricular arrhythmias.
        1) Ventricular premature contractions.
        2) Ventricular tachycardia.
        3) Ventricular fibrillation.
    c. Bradyarrhythmias.
        1) Sinus node dysfunction (bradycardia or sinus arrest).
        2) First-degree AV block.
        3) Second-degree AV block.
        4) Complete AV block (third-degree).
    d. Require no therapy for arrhythmia; or significance of arrhythmia not well known. (May also be classified under other groups—sometimes requiring therapy.)

FURTHER CONSIDERATION OF CLASSIFICATION

In the consideration of arrhythmias, the following factors must also be noted.
1. The cardiac impulse is normally formed in the SA node.
2. The cardiac impulse normally travels from the SA node to atrial muscle to AV node to ventricular muscle.
3. All rhythms that do not originate in the SA node are considered *ectopic* in origin.
4. There may be a disturbance in both cardiac impulse formation and impulse conduction in the same arrhythmia.
5. There is general, but not complete, agreement at present about the relative and the potential danger of most arrhythmias in the presence of acute myocardial infarction.

PRIMARY AND SECONDARY ARRHYTHMIAS

It is important in treating the patient with acute myocardial infarction to distinguish between primary and secondary arrhythmias. This distinction is particularly important from a therapeutic viewpoint.

1. *Primary arrhythmia.* Those arrhythmias occurring in patients without cardiogenic shock or intractable heart failure, and which are likely to be or become a *cause* of serious hemodynamic disturbance in an otherwise "good heart" in the presence of acute myocardial infarction.

2. *Secondary arrhythmias.* Arrhythmias occurring in a patient with established cardiogenic shock or intractable heart failure, being a *result* of the serious disturbance in the hemodynamic state.

Supraventricular Tachycardias (Tachyarrhythmias)

The supraventricular tachycardias include paroxysmal atrial tachycardia, atrial flutter, atrial fibrillation and nodal tachycardia. The guidelines of therapy for each of the supraventricular tachycardias are generally the same.

Atrial fibrillation is the most frequently observed supraventricular tachycardia associated with acute myocardial infarction.[26,140] The other supraventricular tachyarrhythmias also occur in significant numbers. The frequency of occurrence reported depends on the conditions of investigation.

This group usually does not represent the most dangerous of the arrhythmias. The chief hazard is the occurrence of heart failure due to a rapid ventricular response rate.

GOAL OF THERAPY

Almost all undigitalized patients have a ventricular response rate of 120–140, or more, beats/minute with supraventricular tachycardias. The primary goal of therapy is *control of the ventricular rate.* The method of therapy depends on the clinical determination of the patient's current and immediate future tolerance for the rapid ventricular response rate.

Treatment of Supraventricular Tachyarrhythmias

The treatment of supraventricular tachyarrhythmias due to acute myocardial infarction is the administration of *digitalis.* If the patient is in rapidly occurring heart failure, cardioversion may be necessary.

SPECIFICS OF THERAPY

1. If the patient is tolerating the ventricular rate well, IV digitalization should be carried out. For rapid IV digitalization, digoxin,[26,105] ouabain[26] or deslanoside[1,14,25] is used.
   a. Dosage is as follows:
      1) Digoxin (Lanoxin): 0.75 mg. IV initially, followed with 0.25 mg. IV every 1–4 hours until the patient is digitalized.
      2) Strophanthine (ouabain): 0.1 mg. IV approximately every 10–20 minutes, to a total dose of 0.3–0.4 mg. IV in 90 minutes, or 0.7 mg. in 24 hours.
      3) Deslanoside (Cedilanid): 0.8 mg. IV initially, followed by increments of 0.2–0.4 mg. every 1–4 hours to a total of 1.6 mg. or until the desired clinical effect is achieved.
      4) See also Chapter 12.
   b. The digitalizing dose required to achieve an adequate ventricular response in the presence of atrial fibrillation is frequently about 25% greater than that required in the absence of atrial fibrillation. Thus, if atrial fibrillation is converted, manifestations of digitalis toxicity may be seen.[15]
   c. Some authorities feel the dose of digitalis required for digitalization in acute myocardial infarction is about 25% less than that required in the absence of acute myocardial infarction. Thus, particular care is required in the treatment of supraventricular tachyarrhythmias in the presence of acute myocardial infarction so that digitalis toxicity may be avoided.
   d. As supraventricular tachycardias tend to recur in bouts during the first week after acute myocardial infarction, digitalis is probably the preferred therapy initially, reserving electroconversion for the patient who tolerates the arrhythmia poorly or fails to respond to digitalis.

2. If clinical signs of decreased cardiac output (hypotension, increasing congestive failure, oliguria, or ventricular irritability as manifested by VPCs) are obviously developing, then DC precordial shock[26,140] or intracardiac pacing ("overdrive pacing") may be necessary.
   a. A DC countershock of 25 watt-seconds is used, [105,228] increasing to 50, 100, 200 and 400 watt-seconds.
      1) Valium anesthesia (10-20 mg. IV) may be used.[73,105]
   b. If digitalis has previously been administered, protect with lidocaine (Xylocaine) bolus and infusion.

3. If, during digitalization, clinical signs of deterioration appear, electroconversion should be promptly performed.[26,140,263,264]

4. *Maintenance:* After digitalization and maintenance on digitalis, procainamide (500-750 mg. every 4 to 6 hours IM or orally) may be administered if necessary to prevent recurrence. Quinidine sulfate (0.2-0.4 Gm. every 6 hours orally) may also be administered alone or in addition to procainamide to prevent recurrence of supraventricular tachycardias.

a. An adequate dose of digitalis is mandatory before administration of quinidine-like drugs in the presence of supraventricular tachyarrhythmias. Because of the vagolytic effect of these quinidine-like drugs, their use alone or their use in patients who are underdigitalized may lead to rapid ventricular rates (quinidine syncope).

b. See also Digitalis (Chapter 12) and Quinidine (Chapter 9).

5. Methods of increasing vagal stimulation may also be used.
   a. Valsalva maneuver.
   b. Ocular or unilateral carotid pressure.
   c. Digitalize and repeat unilateral carotid pressure.
   d. Edrophonium (Tensilon) in selected instances.

6. Adequate sedation is helpful.

7. Glucose/potassium chloride/insulin "polarizing" solutions have been used but are not generally accepted as helpful in supraventricular tachycardias.

Atrial Premature Contractions

IMPORTANCE IN ACUTE MYOCARDIAL INFARCTION

1. Atrial premature contractions (APCs, PACs) usually indicate dilatation of the atria associated with congestive heart failure. With dilatation there is increased irritability of the atria and increased likelihood of APCs. The occurrence of APCs is frequently observed before any other signs or symptoms of congestive heart failure.

2. APCs are the forerunner of the supraventricular tachyarrhythmias with their associated rapid ventricular response rates. In this regard it should be noted that there is a "vulnerable period" for the atria as well as for the ventricles. It is by the same mechanism that APCs falling on the atrial vulnerable period may cause atrial tachycardia or fibrillation as VPCs cause ventricular tachycardia or ventricular fibrillation (see VPCs, next section).

3. APCs may also result from temporary ischemia of the SA node or portions of the atria.

THERAPY OF APCs

1. Less than 6/minute are of no immediate significance but should be observed closely.

2. If more than 6/minute, or frequent bigeminal or trigeminal APCs are present, it is logical to assume that the probability that a supraventricular tachyarrhythmia will occur is excellent. Therefore the *therapy of choice* for APCs is rapid IV digitalization. The reasons follow.
   a. The inotropic effect of digitalis may correct the congestive heart failure and thus the atrial dilatation that initiates atrial irritability and APCs in some instances.

b. If a supraventricular tachyarrhythmia should occur, the patient will be digitalized or started on digitalis therapy and will, therefore, be protected from the rapid ventricular response rate associated with supraventricular tachyarrhythmias prior to treatment with digitalis. The protection from a rapid ventricular response rate in turn further protects from the occurrence of congestive heart failure.

3. Alternative therapy with quinidine sulfate, 200 mg. every 6 hours, has been suggested, but this is definitely not the initial therapy of choice.

Nodal Premature Contractions

1. Nodal premature contractions (NPCs, PNCs) actually do not arise from the AV node. They arise from the junctional tissue in the atria above (superior) and adjacent to the AV node.

2. As the site of origin of the impulse for NPCs is in the atrium (supraventricular), the significance of NPCs is the same as that of APCs.

3. Criteria for treatment and therapy of NPCs is the same as those for APCs.

Nodal Tachycardia

1. The term "junctional tachycardia" is the scientifically accurate term for nodal tachycardia. This tachycardia actually originates in the junctional tissue lying in the atrium just above (superior) and adjacent to the AV node. Though the terms "junctional tachycardia" and "tachycardia of junctional origin" are scientifically accurate, probably more than 95% of the coronary care units in the country use the term "nodal tachycardia." Therefore, to avoid confusion, junctional tachycardia will be referred to as nodal tachycardia pending the more widespread use of the term denoting its junctional tissue origin.

2. Criteria for treatment and therapy of nodal tachycardia are the same in all aspects as those for other supraventricular tachyarrhythmias.

Hazards of Therapy of Supraventricular Tachyarrhythmias

In patients treated with digitalis and diuretics before admission, the arrhythmia may be due to digitalis intoxication, with or without associated hypokalemia.

1. If supraventricular arrhythmia due to digitalis toxicity is present with acute myocardial infarction, DC precordial shock may be necessary if rapid heart failure and/or altered hemodynamic balance is occurring. Note the danger of digitalis and cardioversion.[263,264]
   a. If cardioversion is *essential*, pretreatment with an antiarrhythmic agent such as lidocaine, via bolus and drip, is essential in order to prevent other serious arrhythmias due to cardioversion.

2. *Remember:* Hazards of electroconversion of digitalis-induced arrhythmias are well known.[263,264] Electroversion of digitalis-induced arrhythmias may cause serious sinus block, AV node dysfunction or ventricular tachycardia or fibrillation.
3. Risks of electroconversion with antiarrhythmic pretreatment must be weighed against permitting the supraventricular tachyarrhythmia to persist while treating digitalis intoxication.
4. Before electroversion in digitalis-induced supraventricular arrhythmias, a pacing electrode is passed into the right ventricle by some clinicians so that adequate heart rate can be maintained if bradycardia occurs.

Ectopic Ventricular Arrhythmias

Ventricular Premature Complexes*

INCIDENCE

Ventricular premature complexes (VPCs) are the commonest arrhythmias observed in patients with acute myocardial infarction, being seen in from 75 to 85% of the patients admitted to coronary care units.

Ventricular premature complexes are important because, under a number of conditions, they have a serious prognostic significance, based on their tendency to cause ventricular tachycardia and ventricular fibrillation. The circumstances under which these life-threatening arrhythmias are particularly apt to occur are the indications for therapy of VPCs. It has been repeatedly noted that ventricular tachycardia and ventricular fibrillation most often occur the first hospital day and are often preceded by ventricular ectopic beats, particularly of the R-on-T type.

INDICATIONS FOR THERAPY

Therapy of VPCs cannot be realistically separated from therapy of other ectopic ventricular arrhythmias.

*References: 3, 5, 26, 31, 37, 50, 97, 242, 258, 259.

Therefore, other aspects of ectopic ventricular arrhythmias generally will be considered here. Because certain circumstances of occurrence of VPCs are apt to trigger ventricular tachycardia and/or ventricular fibrillation, VPCs are treated if the following criteria exist.

1. Occurrence of VPCs (even infrequently) during the first 24 hours after acute myocardial infarction.[259]
2. VPCs occurring more frequently than 5/minute after the first 24 hours following acute myocardial infarction.
3. The VPCs are multifocal. Multifocal or consecutive VPCs carry a more serious prognosis than bigeminal VPCs, though bigeminy is more common.
4. Salvos (runs) of 2 or more VPCs. (*Note:* Ventricular tachycardia is defined as 3 or more consecutive VPCs.)
5. The VPCs show R-on-T interruption (occur in the ventricular vulnerable period).

PATHOLOGIC PHYSIOLOGY OF ECTOPIC VENTRICULAR ARRHYTHMIAS

Premature Ventricular Contractions and the "Vulnerable Period"

1. It has been shown experimentally in ani-

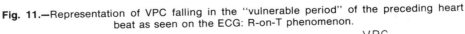

Fig. 11.—Representation of VPC falling in the "vulnerable period" of the preceding heart beat as seen on the ECG: R-on-T phenomenon.

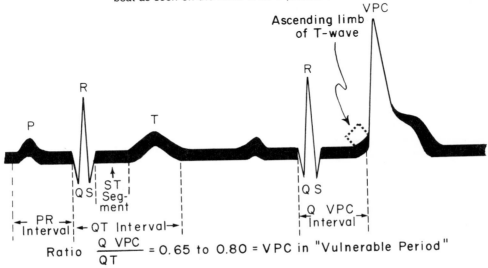

mals[3,30,31] and proved by observation of continuous electrocardiographic monitoring in man[32] that, in the presence of acute myocardial infarction, there is a period in each cardiac cycle that manifests particular susceptibility to ventricular fibrillation if a VPC falls within that period. This period of time in the cardiac cycle is called the "vulnerable period" or, more specifically, the "ventricular vulnerable period." The VPC initiating on the up-slope or apex of the preceding T-wave (R-on-T phenomenon) occurs during this period. In mammals, including man, the vulnerable period is the time, as displayed on the ECG, when the ratio of Q-VPC/QT intervals range from 0.65 to 0.80 (Fig. 11). The duration of the vulnerable period is from 20 to 40 msec.

2. Findings related to the ventricular vulnerable period:

  a. External electrical stimuli, applied experimentally, during the ventricular vulnerable period, can produce ventricular tachycardia or fibrillation if the stimulation is of sufficient intensity.[23] This is true of the normal as well as the acutely injured heart.

    1) The threshold for ventricular fibrillation due to impulses falling in the ventricular vulnerable period is *much less* in the presence of acute myocardial infarction than in the normal heart.

  b. Experimentally and clinically, myocardial ischemia lowers the threshold for ventricular arrhythmias when an external stimulus falls in the ventricular vulnerable period. (*Note:* Caution regarding electric shocks in the coronary care unit.)

  c. In both experimental animals and man, stimuli arising *within the heart* (i.e., VPCs) have also been demonstrated to produce ventricular tachycardia if they occur during the ventricular vulnerable period.[3,23,37]

    1) There is also a vulnerable period for the atria, when stimuli arising in the atria may cause atrial tachycardia or fibrillation.

  d. There is a higher incidence of sudden death in association with VPCs which demonstrate R-on-T phenomenon than in association with VPCs which do not demonstrate this phenomenon.

  e. It has been demonstrated[37] in experimental animals with acute myocardial infarction that there is a vulnerable period for ventricular *tachycardia* during the first week after coronary artery closure which requires only a fraction of the energy necessary to produce ventricular *fibrillation.* Clinically, if not terminated, ventricular tachycardia usually leads to ventricular fibrillation.

Other Related Factors

1. Digitalis in excess dosage has been found to markedly *reduce* the threshold for ventricular tachycardia produced by stimuli falling *outside* the vulnerable period.

2. In acute myocardial infarction, sympathetic stimulation or catecholamines from any source will lower the threshold for ventricular arrhythmias. This fact is important in relation to the therapy of cardiogenic shock[138] and the prevention of untoward anxiety.

Hemodynamics of VPCs

When ventricular contraction is initiated by ectopic impulses, the resulting reduction in cardiac performance is closely related to the *frequency* of the *premature contractions.*[11]

GOAL OF THERAPY

The goal of therapy in ventricular ectopic arrhythmias is to decrease the irritability of the cardiac muscle and thus to decrease the likelihood that VPCs will occur, or if they do occur that they will lead to ventricular tachycardia and/or ventricular fibrillation. Thus, the ultimate purpose of therapy of VPCs in acute myocardial infarction is to decrease the probability of occurrence of these potentially fatal arrhythmias.

THERAPY OF PREMATURE VENTRICULAR CONTRACTIONS

1. Lidocaine (Xylocaine) Initial Drug of Choice

Lidocaine (Xylocaine) in repeated stat doses or via continuous IV drip, or by both methods of IV administration, is the drug of choice in initial therapy of VPCs or nonsustained runs of ventricular tachycardia (6–20 VPCs in sequence).[3,26,105] Dosage is given under Lidocaine Therapy for Ectopic Ventricular Arrhythmias, this section. (See also Lidocaine in Chapter 9.)

2. Procainamide (Pronestyl)

  a. Some physicians use procainamide in stat IV and/or continuous IV drip.

    1- Lidocaine is preferable as initial therapy.

  b. Dose: 50–200 mg. IV stat; IV infusion 25–50 mg./minute maximum.

  c. Other clinicians use lidocaine or procainamide IV, then oral or IM procainamide as maintenance therapy.

3. Route of Administration

When the criteria for therapy of VPCs occur, the IV route of administration of therapeutic agents should be used initially in order to achieve an adequate blood level rapidly. In using lidocaine, a bolus of the drug is necessary to obtain a sustained initial blood level. The same is probably true of procainamide, though initial IV therapy with procainamide *must* be at a rate slower than that for lidocaine since procainamide is more apt to produce severe hypotension.

4. *Procainamide Prophylaxis*[258]
   a. In an excellent double-blind study in patients with acute myocardial infarction, procainamide used before occurrence of *any* arrhythmias was found to be highly effective in decreasing the frequency of all types of ectopic ventricular arrhythmias.[258]
   b. Routine prophylaxis is contraindicated in patients with:
      1) Pulmonary edema or other evidence of severe congestive heart failure.
      2) Cardiogenic shock.
      3) Partial or complete AV block.
      4) Recent cardiac arrest.
      5) History of severe adverse reaction to procainamide.
   c. Dosage
      1) Serum level determinations have revealed that an effective weight dosage level may be rapidly achieved and maintained with the following oral or IM dosage; the loading dose followed by administration every 3 hours (in the absence of congestive heart failure, renal disease, hepatic disease or other contraindications):
         a) Loading dose of 1.0 Gm.
         b) Patient weight less than 120 lb.: give 250 mg. every 3 hours (2 Gm./day).
         c) Patient weight 120–200 lb.: give 375 mg. every 3 hours (3 Gm./day).
         d) Patient weight over 200 lb.: give 500 mg. every 3 hours (4 Gm./day).
      2) Observe for usual signs of cardiac toxicity. Congestive heart failure and kidney and liver diseases affect metabolism of the drug.
      3) Laboratory determinations of plasma concentrations of procainamide are desirable. The therapeutic range in acute myocardial infarction is 4–6 mg./L. of plasma. Higher plasma levels may cause toxicity in the presence of acute myocardial infarction. When it is not possible to obtain plasma measurements, the given dosage schedule will leave some patients unprotected and others intoxicated.

Lidocaine Therapy for Ectopic Ventricular Arrhythmias

INITIAL LIDOCAINE THERAPY

1. Therapy is initiated with a stat dose administered IV, the dose being 1–2 mg./kg. of body weight, given as a bolus. Maintenance therapy with IV lidocaine (1–2 mg./minute) is started immediately.
   a. Often one dose will abolish arrhythmia for 15–20 minutes.

   b. If arrhythmia persists after 3 minutes, administer additional doses of 1 mg./kg. every 3–5 minutes until one of the following occurs:
      1) VPCs disappear.
      2) Total dose of 5 mg./kg. is given over a 15–20 minute period (including infusion). Do not exceed this dose, unless the life-threatening nature of the VPCs is greater than the hazards of lidocaine toxicity. (N.B.: Clinical judgment.)

LIDOCAINE INFUSION MAINTENANCE THERAPY

1. Lidocaine via continuous IV drip is the safest, most rapidly adjustable method.
2. This method of therapy is initiated *immediately* following the initial bolus of lidocaine.
3. The lidocaine drip may be used alone for several days, or therapy with procainamide may be instituted orally or IM and the lidocaine infusion gradually decreased as the procainamide is absorbed.

Suggested Method (for dilutions, see Appendix)

1. Adjust the initial drip rate to deliver 3–5 mg./minute for 15–20 minutes.
2. If VPCs are suppressed, decrease the drip rate by 1 mg./minute every 1 or 2 hours, while continuing to maintain VPC suppression until the patient is weaned from the drug, or:
   a. It may be desirable to maintain the drip at 1–2 mg./minute for 24–48 hours.
   b. It may be desirable to institute maintenance therapy with procainamide before weaning from lidocaine.
3. If at any time the arrhythmia recurs, the drip rate is increased to a level of 3–5 mg./minute or less, to abolish the VPCs.
4. If there is a *sudden* increase in frequency of ectopic ventricular beats, additional 1 mg./kg. stat doses are given via IV bolus.
5. Note: Dosage of over 5 mg./minute (300 mg./hour) is hazardous with regard to central nervous system side effects.

Alternative Methods

1. After lidocaine bolus, infuse 1–2 mg./minute initially and await results. Titrate lidocaine drip to maintain VPC suppression. Maximum infusion of lidocaine is 5 mg./minute.
   a. 5 mg./minute is at borderline of toxic dose in an average 70-kg. man.
2. Immediate IM or oral procainamide therapy, 500–750 mg. every 4–6 hours, may be started if desired, and the infusion of lidocaine decreased, according to the antiarrhythmic effects achieved, until the patient is weaned from lidocaine.

a. This method of therapy is usually, but of course not always, successful.

PROCAINAMIDE MAINTENANCE THERAPY

1. When VPC activity is effectively suppressed, procainamide IM has been used alone for maintenance.
    a. Therapy with procainamide is started before lidocaine is gradually discontinued, in order to provide continuous VPC suppressant coverage.
2. Initially, 500–750 mg. is given every 6 hours. A *smaller dose is rarely effective.*
3. Often, 750 mg. every 4–6 hours is required to suppress VPC activity.
4. Recent investigations suggest that administration at 3-hour intervals may be more effective, the dosage being determined on a weight basis (see Procainamide Prophylaxis under Therapy of Premature Ventricular Contractions).
5. After adequate control is satisfactorily maintained, the oral route may be utilized with the same dosage schedule.
    a. It should be noted that; when administered orally or IM procainamide is not likely to produce hypotensive effects and thus competes favorably with IV lidocaine as a maintenance drug. At this point in maintenance therapy, lidocaine has only the advantage of a more accurate and more transient effect via the IV route of administration.
6. After the arrhythmia is quiescent for several days on oral procainamide, the total dose is progressively decreased by 1 Gm. every 48 hours (500 mg. decrease per 24-hour dosage period).
    a. More rapid schedules for decreasing dosage have been utilized, but careful observation is necessary, with rapid reinstitution of previous effective dosage levels if VPCs recur.
    b. It is desirable to begin tapering the antiarrhythmic drug before discharge from the acute coronary care unit, in order to detect recurrence of frequent VPCs.

COMBINATION DRUG MAINTENANCE THERAPY

It may be necessary to utilize both lidocaine infusion and procainamide by some route of administration to maintain suppression of VPCs or other ectopic ventricular arrhythmia.

1. It is sometimes necessary to utilize lidocaine infusion, procainamide therapy and quinidine therapy in combination to suppress ectopic ventricular activity. If so, the initial quinidine dose is 200 mg. every 6 hours.

QUINIDINE MAINTENANCE THERAPY

1. Quinidine sulfate (orally) is *not* preferred over procainamide as maintenance therapy.
2. It may occasionally control frequent VPCs after failure of procainamide.

3. Initial dose when used alone is 400–500 mg. orally every 4–6 hours.
4. Decrease total dose by 300–400 mg. every 48 hours (150–200 mg. decrease per 24-hour dosage period).

HAZARDS OF THERAPY

1. Hazards of toxicity of the initial and maintenance drugs used. (See individual drugs, Chapter 9.)
2. Hazards of interaction of the antiarrhythmic drugs and any other drugs being administered.

Ventricular Tachycardia[†]

INCIDENCE

The reported incidence of ventricular tachycardia (VT) has varied from 6% to 60% in various series when continuous monitoring is carried out. The wide range of reported incidence is dependent upon the method of ECG monitoring, the criteria for diagnosis, the length of time VT is sustained and the presence or absence of shock.[15,26,137,140,162]

DEFINITION

Ventricular tachycardia is defined by the New York Heart Association as a "succession of 3 or more consecutive ventricular premature systoles occurring usually at the rate ranging from 150 to 250 beats per minute." However, most sources now consider any rate over 100/minute to constitute VT if other criteria are met.[77] Certain cases with rates less than 100/minute may also be considered VT when other criteria are met.[137]

PATHOLOGIC PHYSIOLOGY

1. See Pathologic Physiology of Ectopic Ventricular Arrhythmias; and note Definition of VT.
2. It has been demonstrated that VT may reduce coronary blood flow by 60%, with an accompanying fall in blood pressure, even though the rate of VT is not very rapid. Ventricular tachycardia is, therefore, a potent precipitating cause of hypotension and cardiac failure. (*Recall:* Unfavorable hemodynamics of VPCs is proportionate to the frequency of VPCs, and VT is defined as sequential VPCs.) In some instances, this mechanism is a cause of sudden death.[32]

CAUSES IN ACUTE MYOCARDIAL INFARCTION

1. Primary ventricular tachycardia—following VPCs or self-initiating.
2. Secondary ventricular tachycardia—in terminal phases of cardiogenic shock or pulmonary edema or accompanying other arrhythmias, such as advanced degrees of heart block.
3. Causes other than primary or secondary:

[†]References: 14, 15, 19, 22–24, 26, 32, 73, 77, 113, 114, 137, 139, 140, 162.

a. Following electric shock, used in treatment of patients with arrhythmias, *with or without* the stimulus falling in the ventricular vulnerable period.
b. Stimuli from a properly functioning cardiac pacemaker, particularly in the anoxic heart.
c. Malfunction of a pacemaker, stimulating the ventricles at a rapid rate.
d. Digitalis intoxication.
e. Other drugs have been implicated, particularly:
  1) Quinidine.
  2) Procainamide.
  3) Sympathomimetic amines (epinephrine, norepinephrine, isoproterenol and metaraminol).

GOALS OF THERAPY

The goals of therapy of VT are:
1. To restore functional ventricular rate in the presence of *sustained* ventricular tachycardia.
2. To decrease ventricular irritability in the presence of short, *nonsustained* bursts of ventricular tachycardia.
3. To convert to normally conducted beat for improved hemodynamics.

DIVISION INTO GROUPS FOR PURPOSES OF THERAPY[22–24, 26]

Group I: Short, nonsustained runs of 3 or more consecutive ventricular premature complexes. The patient experiences no significant decrease in cardiac output.
  This is the most commonly observed form of ventricular tachycardia in patients with acute myocardial infarction monitored in the acute coronary care unit.
Group II: This group represents a small group of patients with *sustained ventricular tachycardia* who have *no* signs of *decreased cardiac output.* The patient is normotensive, alert, unaware of any change of heart rate and without congestive heart failure.
Group III: This group consists of patients with *sustained ventricular tachycardia* associated *with* signs of immediate and *severe decreased cardiac output.* It includes most of the patients with sustained ventricular tachycardia.

GROUP I THERAPY OF CHOICE

This group should be treated rapidly, thus preventing occurrence of the more dangerous groups. (*Danger:* This is a forerunner of sustained ventricular tachycardia or ventricular fibrillation.)
1. Initial therapy: Same as for VPCs (pp. 29–30).
2. Maintenance therapy: Same as for VPCs (pp. 30–31).
3. If short runs persist with lidocaine drip of 1–5 mg./minute, it may be necessary to institute some part of the following therapy:
  a. Administer more than a 5 mg./minute dose of lidocaine (hazard of toxicity).

b. Add 500–750 mg. procainamide IM or IV every 4–6 hours; this may permit smaller doses of lidocaine. The IV solution consists of 1 Gm. procainamide in 250 ml. solution (4 mg./ml. of solution). The rate of IV procainamide is not to exceed 25–50 mg./minute at any time; monitor blood pressure.
4. Monitor the ECG and blood pressure during procainamide or lidocaine administration.
5. *Note:* If large doses of antiarrhythmic drugs are required to control ventricular irritability, exclude hypokalemia as a potentiating factor.

GROUP II THERAPY

Drug therapy

1. In this group of patients with sustained VT the characteristics of Group III may develop. Should this occur, immediate cardioversion is indicated.
2. If signs of decreased cardiac output do not occur, initial and maintenance therapy is with lidocaine (Xylocaine) via 2 mg./kg. bolus followed immediately by lidocaine infusion of 2–4 mg./minute for the average 70-kg. man.
3. If lidocaine does not convert the VT, additional drug therapy with procainamide drip (as for Group I) may be instituted, so long as signs of decreased cardiac output have not occurred.
4. Should signs of Group III appear, cardioversion (see below) should be instituted at any point after the steps outlined in number 2 above.
5. Propranolol (Inderal) has been utilized as a supplement for refractory VT. Dosage is 2–3 mg. IV slowly.
  a. Propranolol is a potent and dangerous drug because of its negative inotropic effect. When cardiac function is already compromised, as in VT propranolol should be used only as a last resort.
  b. If propranolol is used at all, it should be as a supplement in refractory cases when cardioversion has already failed.
6. Quinidine supplement, in doses of 0.4 Gm./hour for a few doses only, has been recommended if lidocaine plus procainamide therapy does not effect cardioversion. Quinidine is a hazardous drug and is of questionable value when acute myocardial infarction has occurred.

Cardioversion

1. A DC precordial synchronized shock is used if the arrhythmia is not abolished after drug therapy. Cardioversion may be used in Group II VT at any time after the administration of lidocaine by bolus and continuing infusion.
2. Strength of DC shock range is from 50 to 400 watt-seconds, with a duration of 2.5 msec. Start with 50 watt-seconds, then 100, 200, 400, respectively.[228]

3. When cardioversion is used in therapy of Group II, premedicate with antiarrhythmic drug. Lidocaine is the drug of choice, administered as a bolus followed by continuous infusion.
4. Premedicate with an anesthetic agent:
   a. Thiopental sodium is administered IV to obtund the patient[22,73] via a 1% solution. Dose is 250–400 mg.
   b. Diazepam (Valium) IV in doses of 15–20 mg., given in 60–90 seconds, has proved effective. This agent has not been associated with VPCs as has thiopental sodium.[73]
5. It has been shown that repeated shocks of direct current produce less myocardial damage than alternating current,[139] but for short term use AC is acceptable if it is the only type available.[22,24]

GROUP III THERAPY

Immediate DC Precordial Shock

1. *Note:* Ventricular tachycardia with effective clinical cardiac arrest must be treated immediately with precordial shock.
2. Synchronized shock should be used if at all possible.
3. Premedicate with lidocaine if possible and if time permits.
4. Do not waste precious time with cardiopulmonary resuscitation, drug administration or even synchronization of the electric discharge to the peak of the R-wave, if this is time consuming.
   a. If ventricular fibrillation due to unsynchronized high energy occurs after the first precordial shock, administer a second shock to convert from this arrhythmia.
5. Immediately after successful primary cardioversion from VT, administer a 1–2 mg./kg. stat IV dose of lidocaine (Xylocaine) and start a continuous maintenance drip if lidocaine has not been administered prior to conversion.

Maintenance Therapy

1. After cardioversion and lidocaine infusion therapy, the patient should be maintained on prophylactic procainamide therapy for several weeks.[23]

HAZARDS OF THERAPY

1. Hazards of the antiarrhythmic drugs used. (See individual drugs, Chapter 9.)
2. Hazards of interaction of other drugs with the antiarrhythmic drugs utilized.
3. Hazards of DC precordial synchronized or unsynchronized shock. Also, the other electrical hazards of precordial shock.[114]

ADDITIONAL INFORMATION

1. With VT in the presence of pre-existing complete AV block, synchronized precordial shock is still the therapy of choice.[26,97] Premedicate with lidocaine.
   a. Combination of VT with advanced AV block occurs rather frequently.[87]
   b. If possible, a transvenous catheter pacemaker should be placed before synchronized shock so that electronic pacing may be started immediately if conversion is to complete AV block.[23,97] Time may not permit this procedure.
2. In the presence of acute myocardial infarction, VT is most apt to occur the first day of infarction and with decreasing frequency over the first 2 weeks.[137]

DIGITALIS AND VENTRICULAR TACHYCARDIA

1. Digitalis has been considered to be contraindicated in VT, due to the likelihood of initiating ventricular fibrillation. However, if VT produces heart failure and rapid conversion attempts are unsuccessful, digitalize the patient.[14,23]
2. Do not use quinidine if VT is due to digitalis intoxication. Quinidine may convert to the even more serious ventricular fibrillation.[23]
3. If VT is due to digitalis intoxication, the following drugs may be useful:
   a. Lidocaine (Xylocaine) via 1–2 mg./kg. bolus, followed by infusion of 1–2 mg./minute is rapidly becoming the drug of choice.
   b. Propranolol (Inderal) is given in the usual dose of 0.05–0.1 mg./kg. IV over 2–5 minutes, or 10–30 mg. orally every 6 hours.
   c. Diphenylhydantoin sodium (Dilantin) in a dose of 250 mg. IV over 3–5 minutes has been suggested. The maintenance dose of diphenylhydantoin sodium might be 200–400 mg. orally 2 or 3 times a day. The IV dosage of diphenylhydantoin given before toxic side effects occur depends on the speed of infusion: slow infusion gives few side effects; rapid infusion gives frequent side effects.
      1) Alternate doses given more slowly are also recommended due to toxic side effects of rapid administration. (See Diphenylhydantoin, Chapter 9.)
4. If VT is digitalis induced, and countershock and/or cardiopulmonary resuscitation is necessary, use lidocaine infusion before and during resuscitation.[19]

Ventricular Fibrillation

1. Ventricular fibrillation is commonly preceded by ventricular tachycardia in acute myocardial infarction patients monitored in the coronary care unit.
2. Ventricular fibrillation is *not* self-limiting. Treatment *must* be prompt and definitive.
3. Mortality from ventricular tachycardia or fibrillation as a secondary arrhythmia complicating cardiogenic shock is extremely high, perhaps greater than 70%.

THERAPY

1. Defibrillate immediately. (See also Cardiopulmonary Resuscitation, Chapter 10.)

    a. Do *not* delay for drug therapy or closed chest massage.

    b. If reversion to sinus rhythm occurs in 60 seconds, additional resuscitation measures are rarely required.

2. Administer a 1–2 mg./kg. stat IV dose of lidocaine (Xylocaine) immediately following return to sinus rhythm. Follow with a maintenance infusion of 1–2 mg./minute.

Bradyarrhythmias‡

DEFINITION

Bradyarrhythmias include:

1. Sinus node dysfunction (sinus arrest or sinus bradycardia).
2. First-degree AV block.
3. Second-degree AV block.
4. Third-degree AV block.

    a. With nodal or ventricular escape (nodal or idioventricular rhythm).

    b. With ventricular asystole.

INCIDENCE

1. Patients with acute myocardial infarction, who are continuously monitored in the coronary care unit and who do not show shock, demonstrate about a 25% incidence of some type of bradyarrhythmia.[26,37,156,172]

    a. About one-half have sinus node dysfunction and one-half show advanced heart block.[26,37,172,175]

    b. The reported incidence of all degrees of heart block in acute myocardial infarction is quite variable and averaged about 15% in one review reporting more than 4,700 cases *not monitored* by ECG.[35] The frequency of detection of advanced heart block depends on factors related to ECG monitoring and the stage of therapeutic intervention in the AV block process. The reported incidence appears to be higher when continuous monitoring is carried out.

2. Those patients with acute myocardial infarction who have cardiogenic shock have about an 80% incidence of some form of bradyarrhythmia.[26]

    a. About 15% of these are sinus node dysfunction.

    b. About 85% are advanced heart block.

    c. The mortality rate when cardiogenic shock is complicated by complete AV block was 50–70%[21,26,34,35,117,152] in numerous series of patients studied since the advent of coronary care units and continuous ECG monitoring.

MORTALITY

Total mortality figures reported in patients with acute myocardial infarction and advanced heart block varies, the average being about 40%. About one-half die on the day of admission, and most of the fatalities have occurred by the end of the first week.

GOAL OF THERAPY

The goal of therapy is to *maintain an adequate ventricular rate*. The deleterious effect of a slow heart rate on a diseased heart which may have a fixed stroke volume is well known.[119] Increasing the heart rate will frequently improve cardiac output. Therefore, maintenance of an adequate ventricular rate is the goal of therapy in bradyarrhythmias.

Acute AV block following acute myocardial infarction is usually temporary. The combination of a low cardiac output, myocardial hypoxia from a slow heart rate and a damaged, irritable myocardium often predisposes to the potential dangers of (1) prolonged asystole, resulting in syncope and death, or (2) the onset of ectopic ventricular tachyarrhythmias.[21,35] Therefore, if the cardiac output can be maintained through the period of acute block until the return of normal rhythm, the outlook is improved. The duration of complete heart block varies, the mean in one study being 2½ days.[174]

Most authorities feel the "critical rate" is about 50 beats/minute. It is felt that therapy should be instituted to prevent the patient from falling below this critical rate, or that therapy should be instituted as promptly as possible should this rate be reached. It must be remembered that the critical rate varies among individuals. Maximum cardiac output is usually achieved between 60 and 75 beats/minute.

The current effective methods for treating bradyarrhythmias complicating acute myocardial infarction include the use of atropine, of dilute solutions of sympathomimetic amines (isoproterenol) and of transvenous intracardiac pacing. An adequate heart rate and cardiac output are essential, and persistent bradyarrhythmias complicating acute myocardial infarction have long been regarded as a poor prognostic sign.

During the presence of a bradyarrhythmia, the myocardial infarction and its other complications are treated in the usual manner, except that when advanced heart block is present, digitalis, lidocaine, procainamide and quinidine may be contraindicated, since these drugs depress impulse formation in the AV node as well as conduction through the junctional tissues, AV node and ventricles.

‡References: 3, 13–15, 20, 21, 25–27, 32, 34, 35, 37, 87, 105, 117, 119, 140, 143–145, 147–150, 152, 156, 166, 172–175, 257.

If an artificial pacemaker is inserted, antiarrhythmic drugs may be used as otherwise indicated.[34,35] The drug most usually used to combat ectopic ventricular arrhythmias associated with bradyarrhythmias is lidocaine (Xylocaine) given IV as a 1-2 mg./kg. bolus, followed by a 1-2 mg./minute IV drip, with dosage increased as necessary.

PATHOLOGIC PHYSIOLOGY

1. Bradyarrhythmias are frequently associated with diaphragmatic (inferior) myocardial infarcts. The volume of ventricular myocardial damage is rarely large in diaphragmatic myocardial infarction, making the ultimate prognosis for the patient who survives the acute phase of infarction quite good.[13] However, the acute phase of diaphragmatic (inferior, posterior) myocardial infarction is hazardous, principally because in 90% of instances, it is right coronary occlusion which results in diaphragmatic infarcts, and there is almost always an associated ischemia of the AV node and the His bundle with right coronary occlusion.[13,35]

2. In the presence of right coronary artery occlusion, pathologic and coronary angiographic studies have disclosed that there is rarely actual occlusion of the smaller arterial branch to the AV node or necrosis of the AV node or bundle of His. Therefore, the advanced heart block associated with this clinical situation is due to potentially reversible ischemia and not necrosis. It could be anticipated—and is in fact clinically correlated—that complete heart block following right coronary arterial occlusion and diaphragmatic infarction will subside spontaneously if the patient survives for more than a few days.[35]

3. It has also been noted that Mobitz type I (Wenckebach) second-degree AV block seen with *inferior* (diaphragmatic, posterior) *infarction* and associated with *reversible ischemia* of the AV node is seen with right coronary artery occlusion. This block carries a better prognosis than does the Mobitz type II second-degree block associated with an infra AV node *necrosing lesion* of the bifurcation or bundle branches seen with occlusion of a branch of the left coronary artery and *anterior infarction*.[273]

   Because of the irreversible lesion mentioned above, complete (antegrade) AV block (i.e., complete heart block) with slow, unstable idioventricular pacemaker is seen with anteroseptal infarction.

4. It has been shown that in advanced AV block, anterior infarcts (representing 25% of the total) or inferior infarcts (representing 55%) are present in 80% of instances, the balance being represented by subendocardial infarcts or nonclassifiable infarcts.[87]

5. Over half the right coronary occlusions are also associated with ischemia and/or infarction of the SA node. This occurs because the artery to the SA node comes from the right coronary artery in 50% of instan-

ces. It can thus be easily seen that diaphragmatic (inferior) myocardial infarction would be expected to have, and in fact does have, a definite association with sinus bradycardia and all grades of heart block.[20,25,32,87,105,172,173,175]

6. In fatal cases of advanced heart block, postmortem studies often reveal that there is multiple coronary artery disease; usually with previous infarction in the other portion of the blood supply serving the AV node and His bundle.[13,174]

7. The patient with heart block as a complication of acute myocardial infarction is usually older and probably has had a prior infarct (i.e., multiple coronary artery disease).[13,174]

8. The onset of advanced heart block is nearly always early in the course of acute myocardial infarction, usually on the first day and almost always before the end of the first week.[35] (See pattern of AV block below.)

9. Complete heart block may be associated with a supraventricular (narrow) QRS complex or with an idioventricular (wide) QRS complex. If an idioventricular complex is present, the electrocardiographic diagnosis of acute myocardial infarction may not be possible.

PATTERN OF AV BLOCK IN ACUTE MYOCARDIAL INFARCTION

Development of Advanced AV Block

The establishment of advanced AV block in acute myocardial infarction can be fairly well divided into 3 groups.[87]

1. The group in which advanced AV block apparently develops soon after onset of myocardial damage. These patients present initially with advanced AV block.
   a. This group constitutes about 40-60% of patients manifesting advanced AV block with acute myocardial infarction.[35,87]

2. The group which initially has normal sinus rhythm, but with intraventricular conduction disturbances:
   a. Included are about 20% of those who manifest advanced AV block after acute myocardial infarction.[35,87]
   b. Intraventricular conduction disturbances consist of right, left or bilateral bundle branch block.
   c. Sudden changes to third-degree AV block and cardiac arrest are frequently seen in this group.[87] When mortality is studied as a function of bundle branch block as an isolated factor, there seems to be a high mortality rate of about 60%.[32]

3. The group with neither AV nor intraventricular conduction abnormalities, in which advanced AV block develops progressively over 1-3 days.[87]
   a. This group follows a fairly consistent progression to advanced AV block as follows: Sinus bradycardia—prolonged PR interval—second-degree AV block—complete AV block with nodal pacemaker—

superimposition of right, left or bilateral bundle branch block patterns—slow idioventricular rhythm.

b. It constitutes about 20% of those who manifest advanced AV block with acute myocardial infarction.[87]

Duration of Advanced AV Block

This is highly variable in surviving patients and ranges from a few minutes to persistence following recovery from acute myocardial infarction in an occasional instance.

1. If AV block is persistent following recovery, a permanent implanted demand pacemaker may be needed at a later time.

Regression from Advanced AV Block

Return to normal AV conduction is slow and progressive in most instances, occurring as follows: Third-degree block—second-degree block—transient left or right bundle branch block, or intraventricular conduction defects—PR prolonged—normal sinus rhythm.[87]

Associated Arrhythmias

These are seen under the following specific conditions.

1. Before starting drugs or artificial pacing:
   a. Ventricular tachycardia occurs rather frequently in combination with advanced AV block.[87]
   b. Paroxysmal supraventricular arrhythmias occasionally are seen,[35,87] but are of little clinical significance.

2. After starting isoproterenol (without pacing), several arrhythmias may be seen. These are usually ectopic ventricular arrhythmias and are frequently due to the IV infusion of isoproterenol.[34,35,87]
   a. In this situation use lidocaine therapy to suppress ectopic ventricular arrhythmias while continuing regulated isoproterenol dosage for the AV block.

3. During artificial pacing:
   a. Periods of competition at time of re-establishment of sinus rhythm if a fixed-rate pacemaker is being used. Demand-type pacemakers usually avoid this problem.
   b. VPCs: The usual treatment of VPCs effectively controls this arrhythmia.
   c. Ventricular tachycardia: Use of DC electric shock, followed by drug maintenance therapy usually effectively controls this arrhythmia.
   d. Any arrhythmia seen with the insertion of the transvenous pacemaker electrode.

Sinus Node Dysfunction

The conditions included are sinus bradycardia, at a rate of 50 beats/minute or less, and sinus arrest with escape rhythm or ventricular asystole.

THERAPY

Atropine

Atropine is the drug of choice for sudden episodes, particularly for sinus bradycardia if cardiogenic shock is absent.[14,26,35,173]

1. Dose of 0.3–2 mg. IV, given over several minutes, improves function in most instances.[14,20,26] Frequent 0.3 mg. increments to a total dose of 2 mg. may be used.
2. Onset of atropine effect occurs in 2–3 minutes.[20,26]
3. Duration of action is usually 2–4 hours.[20,26]
4. Dose may be repeated if bradycardia and hypotension recur,[20] the dose being given every 3 or 4 hours.
5. Atropine has also been used when bradycardia is associated with low atrial pacemaker site and nodal rhythm, that is, nodal bradycardia. Beneficial results are seen in heart rate, arterial blood pressure and general clinical state.[20]
6. Atropine is not recommended for maintenance, because the drug:
   a. Almost invariably produces urinary retention.
   b. May precipitate acute glaucoma.
   c. May precipitate mental aberration and, in some instances, actual psychosis.

Isoproterenol

1. If there is no response to atropine, use an IV infusion of isoproterenol (4 mg./L. dextrose in water equals 4 μg./ml.). Use a microdrop infusion set.[26]
2. Adjust rate of administration to provide a normal sinus rate, usually of 60 beats/minute or more, or until toxic effects of the drug are noted.
3. Start drip at 1.25 ml./minute (5 μg./minute). Watch for toxic effects.
   a. Some authorities suggest 1 mg./500 ml. of 5% D/W, (2 μg./ml.) for better control and avoidance of overdose.[173,175]
4. Lidocaine (Xylocaine) is given to suppress ectopic rhythms seen with isoproterenol (Isuprel). Have lidocaine drip attached to patient's IV tubing in readiness.

Atrial Pacing

Although most authorities do not insert an electrode pacing catheter for sinus node dysfunction unless drug therapy is ineffective, some[26] feel the safest method of therapy is via transvenous intracardiac pacing of the right atrium.

1. Indications for atrial pacing are based on a clinical estimation of the patient's tolerance for a slow heart rate and the effectiveness of drug therapy.[26,156] VPCs, progressive cardiac decompensation, angina pectoris, decreased cerebral blood flow and frank shock are

felt to be definite indications for a therapeutic trial of atrial pacing.

2. Atrial pacing avoids the hazard of inducing ventricular tachycardia or fibrillation with isoproterenol.
3. *Note:* It is difficult to get consistent atrial capture with currently available intracardiac electrodes.
4. Often the pacing catheter slips across into the right ventricle, therefore not maintaining contact with the atrial wall.
5. If atrial pacing is not reliable, yet pacing is clearly indicated, the electrode may be advanced into the right ventricle.[26,156]

First-Degree AV Block

THERAPY

1. Usually none—by most authorities.
2. Some clinicians prophylactically insert an intracardiac electrode into the right ventricle[26] of patients receiving myocardial depressant drugs or digitalis.
   a. The patient is *not* paced.
   b. The electrode is electively passed to insure control of heart rate should a more advanced AV block suddenly occur.

Second-Degree AV Block

THERAPY

1. Initially give IV atropine[26,175] in dosage as for sinus node dysfunction.
2. Isoproterenol (Isuprel) via IV drip is used in the following situations:
   a. When no response to atropine occurs.
   b. If clinical condition is deteriorating despite atropine.
   c. As maintenance following initial atropine therapy.
      1) It is used as continued maintenance when inferior (posterior, diaphragmatic) infarction is present and therapeutic response is adequate. (Usually associated with Mobitz type I second-degree AV block.)
      2) It is used as temporary maintenance when anterior infarction (associated with Mobitz type II second-degree AV block) is present, while the transvenous electrode catheter is being inserted and until artificial cardiac pacing is required.
3. Lidocaine (Xylocaine) infusion should be attached and ready for use should isoproterenol produce ectopic ventricular activity.

Cardiac Pacing

The necessity for artificial cardiac pacing in the presence of second-degree AV block depends on the location of the infarction. In inferior wall infarction, artificial pacing is not usually necessary. In anterior wall infarction pacing is frequently required.

1. Most instances of second-degree AV block associated with *inferior* (posterior, diaphragmatic) *wall infarction* are Mobitz type I (Wenckebach) blocks that do not require artificial pacing. Treatment is with IV isoproterenol if the ventricular rate falls below 50 or hemodynamic deterioration occurs.
   a. In instances of Mobitz type I AV block with ventricular rate less than 50 and no response to isoproterenol (particularly with VPCs or frank shock), a transvenous electrode catheter must be placed and artificial pacing instituted.
2. Most instances of second-degree AV block associated with *anterior wall infarction* are Mobitz type II blocks. This rare type of AV block carries a poor prognosis, and early insertion of transvenous pacing electrode for standby purposes is suggested.
   a. Therapy with isoproterenol is given before and during insertion of the pacing electrode, with lidocaine infusion attached for use if necessary.

PROGNOSIS

Second-degree heart block in the absence of cardiogenic shock may be satisfactorily treated as outlined here, with a low incidence of cardiac arrest. The occurrence of third-degree block will alter this prognosis considerably.

MOBITZ TYPES I AND II SECOND-DEGREE AV BLOCKS

It is important to distinguish between the 2 types of second-degree AV block in the presence of acute myocardial infarction because the underlying pathology, clinical significance and method of acute treatment differs for each type of block.

Mobitz Type I Block

Mobitz type I block (Wenckebach block or phenomenon) consists of a block proximal to the bundle of His. Electrocardiographic diagnosis may be made by any of the following:

1. Wenckebach phenomenon (progressive PR lengthening until a ventricular complex is dropped).
2. Transition from or to a lesser degree of AV block.
3. Transition to AV dissociation with occasional ventricular captures.
4. Comparison of the PR intervals of the conducted beats or of the captures in the same record will reveal the expected variations of PR interval in type I block.

Mobitz Type II Block

"This type of block is characterized by failure of a ventricular response, without antecedent progressive lengthening of AV conduction time....In its more advanced form several consecutive atrial impulses are blocked, giving rise to high degree partial block and to intermittent periods of prolonged ventricular asystole." [273]

1. Electrocardiographic determination of Mobitz type II block is made on the basis of a PR interval in the conducted beat which is stable (constant) with 2:1 or greater constant AV block.

Complete AV Block (Third-Degree Block)

GOAL OF THERAPY

The goal of therapy is to *maintain an adequate ventricular rate*. Methods to achieve this goal vary with the clinical situation. Since there is usually an associated nodal or idioventricular escape rhythm at a rate of 35–40 beats/minute, immediate therapy must be begun.

1. As pervenous insertion of a pacing electrode takes 20–30 minutes under ideal circumstances but pacing is probably the ultimate choice of therapy in the presence of complete heart block, drugs are used *initially* to maintain an adequate ventricular rate while transvenous pacing electrode catheter insertion is accomplished. Drugs alone are used by some clinicians.

THERAPY

1. Initially begin with an IV infusion of isoproterenol (Isuprel), giving 2 mg. in 500 ml. 5% D/W (4 μg./ml.) by means of a microdrop infusion set. This infusion should be administered while an electrode pacing catheter is inserted to carry out demand pacing as the basic form of therapy for third-degree (complete) AV block.
   a. Attempt to speed the heart rate to about 55/minute by varying the rate of drip or by increasing the concentration of isoproterenol.
   b. Maintain attached standby lidocaine drip for use if ectopic ventricular activity occurs due to the third-degree block or isoproterenol therapy.
   c. Some authorities feel this therapy is sufficient unless it is not effective or unless the clinical hemodynamic situation deteriorates.[3,147]
      1) It is an unfortunate fact that up until the present adequate achievement of heart rate has not apparently altered the high over-all statistical mortality rate in this group of patients. However most investigators feel there are specific instances when electrode placement and pacing have been lifesaving.
2. Some authorities initially administer atropine in dosages the same as those for sinus node dysfunction.[20,26]

Artificial Cardiac Pacing§

1. This is considered by most clinicians the preferred

§References: 15, 20, 26, 34, 35, 87, 140, 172, 174, 175, 257.

therapy for third-degree AV block and should be instituted as rapidly as possible.

2. Use a demand-type pacemaker, as this reduces the competition and interference between the natural and the artificially induced beats. This competition is itself capable of producing arrhythmias under the proper circumstances,[27] particularly with a fixed-rate pacemaker.
3. Adjust the heart rate to 75–80 beats/minute.
4. Occasionally it may be necessary to pace the heart at rates of 90–100 beats/minute.
5. Pacing is continued until AV conduction has improved and a normal heart rate is consistently maintained with the pacemaker turned off.
   a. Pacing is continued by some clinicians for at least 3 weeks,[20] since AV block may recur some days after recovery of normal conduction. However, most clinicians pace for shorter periods after recovery of AV conduction.
6. Pathologic physiology of artificial pacing for complete heart block in the presence of acute myocardial infarct: It has been found in a study of a small number of patients with long-standing AV block that cerebral blood flow is significantly decreased and that moderate slowing of the electroencephalogram (EEG) may occur when AV block is of chronic duration.[166] After artificial pacing was instituted in these instances of chronic AV block, cerebral blood flow increased and the EEG improved. These changes paralleled the clinical improvement which accompanied pacemaker therapy.

It would be extremely difficult to do similar studies in acute myocardial infarction with acutely occurring AV block, as institution of rapid therapy is essential to maintain life. Clinically, stupor occurs almost immediately and is corrected when the heart rate is increased, thus indicating that increased cerebral blood flow accompanies the increased heart rate.

Artificial pacing, with increased heart rate, may result in a return to a relatively normal clinical state, or it may have essentially no results if "pump failure" is present.

Other Therapy

1. Corticosteroids are used in the treatment of heart block[105,143,144,148,149] and are routinely used by some clinicians in therapy of AV block. Beneficial effects of the steroids are related to the acceleration of AV conduction or the tendency to reduce serum potassium. They are seldom employed to treat heart block currently because of the greater effectiveness of other forms of therapy, such as isoproterenol and cardiac pacing.
2. Potassium, glucose and insulin combinations are used by some clinicians in the therapy of heart block complicating acute myocardial infarction.[145,150] This

therapy is also not widely used because more dependable therapeutic tools are available.

PROGNOSIS

In the presence of advanced heart block, there is a high incidence of other complications if the patient is on medical therapy alone. Particularly prone to occur are unexpected ventricular arrhythmias or asystole.[172]

Complete heart block is associated with a high mortality rate. This unfortunate circumstance is true whether complete heart block is the result of cardiogenic shock or occurs in the absence of pre-existing cardiogenic shock. The high mortality rate occurs despite the successful treatment of slow heart rates.[20,26,35,140]

Advanced heart block is usually associated with extensive septal involvement and is certainly more apt to occur in the presence of multiple coronary artery disease.

In the presence of advanced heart block, anterior infarcts are associated with a higher mortality rate than are diaphragmatic infarctions, and idioventricular (wide) QRS complexes are associated with a higher mortality than are supraventricular (narrow) QRS complexes.[35]

CHAPTER 5

Cardiogenic Shock*

It is unfortunate that the availability of the intensive coronary care unit has not appreciably altered the prognosis for patients after the clinical features of shock have become manifest.[11] Despite all the therapy now available, shock is responsible for the major proportion of in-hospital deaths due to acute myocardial infarction.[158]

It will be one of the major tasks for the future of coronary care to attempt to improve the prognosis for patients with acute myocardial infarction who have manifested the clinical syndrome of shock.

Definition

With cardiogenic shock there is a relatively sudden and sharp reduction in cardiac output. This *decreased cardiac output* is the primary pathologic change and the causative factor in producing the clinical syndrome of cardiogenic shock.[16,42,71,122,130,133,160,179] When the heart fails to function effectively as a contractile pumping mechanism, there is a failure to pump blood into the aorta in sufficient volume and under sufficient pressure to maintain pressure–flow relationships. With decreased aortic pressure there is a stimulation of the aortic and carotid baroreceptors, causing activation of the sympathetic nervous system. With sympathetic activation, norepinephrine and epinephrine are released in order to increase the peripheral vascular resistance (reflex vasoconstriction). This sympathetic activation is the body's normal adjustment mechanism in its attempt to re-establish an adequate pressure-flow relationship, and thus adequate tissue perfusion. For adequate tissue perfusion to exist, an adequate blood supply must reach the arteries, and thus the capillaries, of the tissues. A head of pressure in the arteries is necessary for capillary circulation. The capillary loop is the most important site of tissue perfusion. Adequate tissue perfusion is essential to maintain adequate tissue metabolism.

Adequate tissue metabolism is essential in order to maintain life. An adequate blood flow perfusing the tissue is more important than the blood pressure reading. Hypotension is a *secondary* manifestation of shock.

Hypotension is a symptom of the cardiogenic shock syndrome and is *secondary* to decreased cardiac output. It has been demonstrated in experimental cardiogenic shock[130] that an increase in peripheral resistance to combat the shock syndrome is accompanied by a significant decrease in regional blood flow to the viscera (intestinal, hepatic and renal). The brain and heart are preferentially spared from this increased resistance during cardiogenic shock and consequently receive a larger share of cardiac output. Although a reflex peripheral vasoconstriction (increased peripheral resistance) usually follows decreased cardiac output, peripheral resistance is not always increased in cardiogenic shock. In some patients peripheral resistance may remain unchanged or be lowered. Reflex vasoconstriction with cardiogenic shock is particularly likely to be absent in elderly patients, some diabetics and patients with idiopathic autonomic nervous system disease.

Clinical Recognition

The clinical symptoms and signs of the shock syndrome may include any combination of the following.[11,16,42,130,133,160]

1. Agitation and apprehension, which may be the first signs of impending shock.
2. Hypotension.
3. Small or decreased pulse pressure.
4. Tachycardia.
5. Skin signs: pallor, coldness, moistness (pale, cold, clammy skin).
6. Altered mental status (restlessness, confusion, stupor).
7. Oliguria (decreased urine output).
8. Collapsed superficial veins.
9. Slow capillary filling.

*References 11, 42, 71, 75, 98, 122–125, 131–136, 140, 158–160, 178–181, 183, 253, 256, 260, 262.

LABORATORY MEASUREMENTS

1. Low cardiac output.
2. Increased or normal central venous pressure.
3. Variable values for total peripheral resistance.
4. Lactic acidosis.
5. Hypercapnia.
6. Hypoxia.

These laboratory measurements may depend on the degree and the stage of shock.

INCIDENCE

The incidence of cardiogenic shock complicating acute myocardial infarction is 10–15%.[11,158]

MORTALITY

The mortality associated with treated cardiogenic shock associated with acute myocardial infarction is variably reported as 50–90%.[132,178]

Pathologic Physiology

MYOCARDIAL CONTRACTILITY

Acute myocardial infarction affects the heart's ability to function effectively as a pump. Myocardial contractility is always reduced to some extent following acute myocardial infarction, whether or not cardiogenic shock is present. If contractility is reduced so much that the capability of the injured heart to maintain adequate cardiac output is compromised, arterial blood pressure may be reduced. (See also Chapter 3.)

The left ventricle is well designed to serve as an efficient high-pressure pump, supplying the necessary power to eject blood into the high-pressure and high-resistance systemic circulation circuit in normal circumstances.[11] The left ventricular cavity resembles a cylinder from a functional viewpoint. The circular bundles of heart muscle form a functional cylinder and provide the primary mechanical force for cardiac pumping. During systole, the long axis of the chamber is somewhat shortened. However, the *primary power* for ejection comes from the reduction in diameter of the functional cylinder that composes the left ventricle. Following acute myocardial infarction there is a disruption in the total integrity of the circular muscle bundles, and the mechanical efficiency of the system is greatly reduced. Since the cavity of the left ventricle resembles a cylinder, it has a relatively small surface area. After infarction, muscle tonus of the infarcted area is lost, and during systole the infarcted area balloons outward. In these circumstances the normally small surface area of the ventricular cavity is enlarged, optimal mechanical configuration is disturbed, and power is dissipated in ballooning the infarcted area outward during systole. It appears, therefore, that it is (1) the disrupted continuity of the circular muscle bundles and (2) the local mechanical defect of the infarcted area which account for a sharp decline in the efficiency of ejection, and not the reduction of total viable myocardial area.

CARDIAC OUTPUT

With the decrease in myocardial contractility there is a decrease in the mechanical performance of the heart. With decreased mechanical performance the cardiac output is diminished and the volume of ventricular ejection (stroke volume) may be reduced to levels of approximately one-third normal after onset of shock in man. The period of systolic ejection is also shortened, and power developed by the heart is greatly decreased. Ventricular function may be further compromised by temporary mitral valvular insufficiency due to ischemia of the papillary muscles of the left ventricle.[11]

The major primary component in cardiogenic shock is depressed left ventricular function with decreased cardiac output. The depressed left ventricular function must also be related to a failure of adequate nutrient delivery to the myocardium, either or both physical and biochemical damage to the myocardium and dysfunction in the excitation-contraction coupling mechanism.[133]

Studies in man have revealed that patients in cardiogenic shock have cardiac outputs significantly lower than a similar group of patients with acute myocardial infarction who are not in shock.[179] Cardiac output following acute myocardial infarction is typically decreased to levels 60–80% of normal. In patients who manifest clinical signs of shock there is a much sharper decline, and cardiac output and stroke volume usually decrease to levels 30–50% of normal. The severity of manifest cardiogenic shock corresponds to the relative decrease in cardiac output.[11] The prognosis in cardiogenic shock seems related to the severity of the heart failure.[179]

Decreases in cardiac output comparable to those seen in cardiogenic shock may be observed after acute myocardial infarction in the absence of clinical shock.[11,71] This is possible and is observed because important compensatory changes occur in the peripheral circulation, especially in the venous capacitance circuit.

It is surprising that reduction in work capacity of the heart after acute myocardial infarction is not usually followed by physiologic changes of cardiac failure. In addition, cardiac enlargement, auscultatory or radiographic signs of pulmonary edema and increase in central venous pressure are not consistently observed in patients with cardiogenic shock after acute myocardial infarction, as might be expected. The absence of increased central venous pressure and central congestion is evidence that there are concurrent changes in the peripheral vascular circuit. Presumably, the capacitance of the peripheral circuit increases so that the volume of blood returned to the right heart does not exceed the output of the left ventricle even in the presence of decreased cardiac output. The central venous pressure in cardiogenic shock does not usually reflect the left ventricular pressure.

The occurrence of shock or the degree of shock does not necessarily correspond to the size of the myocardial infarct. The size of infarct does not necessarily measure the severity of the disturbance in the chemical and physiologic process of the heart muscle or the severity of the neurogenic or hemodynamic reactions of the body to the myocardial infarction.[71]

CORONARY BLOOD FLOW

In experimental animal studies, coronary artery flow has been shown to be pressure dependent. When the pressure head is increased, coronary flow is increased. Increased aortic pressure is associated with increases in coronary blood flow. Clearly, aortic pressure and coronary perfusion pressure are important determinants of myocardial function. As the aortic pressure is increased and coronary blood flow improves, performance of the heart improves by way of increases in cardiac output, myocardial oxygen consumption and myocardial lactate consumption.[11] It is this aortic pressure–coronary blood flow relationship that is augmented by certain mechanical aids (e.g., a balloon in the aorta) currently under investigation for use in certain instances of cardiogenic shock.

In experimental coronary occlusion, with coronary angiography, it is thought that vasoconstriction occurred in both the occluded coronary arteries and the non-occluded coronary arteries.[71]

SYMPATHETIC NERVOUS SYSTEM AND PERIPHERAL RESISTANCE

The common denominator in cardiogenic shock is hyperactivity of the sympathetic division of the autonomic nervous system.[133] During clinical shock many of the manifestations of sympathetic nervous system hyperactivity are obvious.[160] With decreased cardiac output there is a fall in the blood pressure in the aorta. With this central aortic pressure decrease there is an activation of the sympathetic nervous system as a physiologic response to counteract or prevent cardiogenic shock. The sympathetic nervous system activation represents the body's attempt to maintain systemic blood pressure by generalized vasoconstriction. The vasoconstriction involves arterioles, arteries, veins and the cardiac chambers.[160]

It is generally agreed that catecholamines in the tissue and plasma are significantly increased with the onset of shock, and this finding has been confirmed both experimentally in animals and clinically in man. It is generally considered that this increase in catecholamines is due to the greatly increased activity of the sympathetic (adrenergic) nervous system.

Sympathetic stimulation activated by the onset of cardiogenic shock results in excesses of endogenous,

and sometimes the therapeutic presence of exogenous, adrenergic (sympathomimetic) amines. This excess of sympathomimetic amines tends to provoke premature ventricular contractions and ventricular tachycardia. It has been demonstrated experimentally that the risk of such arrhythmias is reduced if the tissue catecholamine concentration is depleted by prior treatment with reserpine.[11] Many hypertensive patients have been treated with reserpine and other tissue catecholamine-depleting drugs before the occurrence of acute myocardial infarction.

The vasoconstriction associated with sympathetic activity in cardiogenic shock is sometimes intense. The effect of continued intense vasoconstriction is sometimes deleterious, in that there may be diminished vasoconstrictor response because of anoxia and acidosis. This may be followed by a vicious cycle of diminished vasoconstrictor response and increasing anoxia and acidosis, progressing to the stage of irreversible shock.

There is current increased awareness of the importance of tissue perfusion in the therapy of cardiogenic shock. Therefore, debate of the value of vasodilator versus vasoconstrictor drugs in shock therapy occurs.

PERIPHERAL ARTERIAL RESISTANCE WITH ACUTE MYOCARDIAL INFARCTION

In experimental and clinical studies the peripheral arterial resistance following acute myocardial infarction is more often observed to be increased or within normal limits than to be decreased.[11] There is general agreement that peripheral arterial resistance is not usually decreased following acute myocardial infarction complicated by cardiogenic shock, but the concept has developed that there is *failure of compensatory increase* of resistance in those patients who show no measurable net increase in peripheral arterial resistance. Since catecholamine secretion is characteristically elevated following acute myocardial infarction, failure of end-organ response to the catecholamines rather than absence of adrenergic hormone is theorized. It must be noted that systemic vascular resistance as measured clinically has varied considerably in patients with acute myocardial infarction.[11,71,133-135,159,179] This may be due to variable vasoconstrictor responsiveness due to variable degrees of anoxia and acidosis of the tissues (i.e., the failure of end-organ response noted above).

When increased peripheral arterial resistance occurs, it is thought that the reflex response to low arterial pressure is mediated through stimulation of the carotid and aortic baroreceptors. This results in the outpouring of catecholamines (norepinephrine and epinephrine) from the sympathetic nerve endings and adrenal medulla. This increase in circulating and tissue levels of catecholamines causes vasoconstriction in the adrenergically sensitive splanchnic, renal and cutaneous beds. The vasoconstriction then produces the classic clinical signs of pale, cold, moist skin and reduced urinary output.

This redistribution of blood flow allows for preferential perfusion of the heart and brain, nature's way of preserving life.[135]

CAPACITANCE (MICROCIRCULATION)

Capacitance represents the capacity of the vascular system to store and withhold the intravascular components from active circulation. Capacitance is definitely affected by shock and by the sympathetic nervous system stimulation associated with cardiogenic shock.

Arterioles determine outflow resistance from the heart and are termed resistance vessels. Capillaries and veins determine capacity and are termed capacitance vessels.

The resistance vessels (arterioles) contain alpha adrenergic receptors sensitive to neural discharges, epinephrine and norepinephrine and vasodilator beta receptors sensitive to epinephrine.

The capacitance vessels (capillaries and veins) are considered to have only alpha receptors, and contraction of these vessels may persist longer than that of resistance vessels, leading to stagnant blood flow, escape of fluid into extravascular spaces, aggregation of blood elements, sludging and even thrombosis.

The release of potent vasoconstrictors at sympathetic nerve endings in association with cardiogenic shock results in pre- and postcapillary vasoconstriction in the cutaneous and visceral microcirculation, with a net increase in total peripheral resistance. Increases in the viscosity of the blood add to resistance of flow in the microcirculation.[130]

In the presence of cardiogenic shock, major capacitance changes occur in the venous and capillary beds. Substantial increases in cardiac output are frequently observed if plasma expansion is undertaken during shock.[262] It appears that loss of effective volume occurs in part due to pooling of blood in the venous-capillary capacitance circuit. This pooling of blood in turn further reduces cardiac output.

Changes in capacitance appear to be secondary to the initial myocardial injury and subsequent chain of events in cardiogenic shock, but they may account for the continuing reduction in cardiac output and the appearance of further clinical features of severe and irreversible shock.

In experimental animals, after coronary thrombosis, there is a progressive reduction in blood volume over a period of 5 hours. The reduction in volume follows rather than accompanies the onset of clinical shock. This would seem to correlate with changes in capacitance which may increase the severity of cardiogenic shock after its onset.

METABOLIC CHANGES IN CARDIOGENIC SHOCK

In the "low perfusion state" there is not adequate oxygen to meet the requirements of tissues. The conversion of pyruvate to carbon dioxide and water is sup-pressed or arrested and anaerobic metabolism occurs, with an excess of lactate accumulating in the tissues and subsequently in the blood stream. There is also an outpouring of lactate from the ischemic heart. However, the large increases in lactate concentration in arterial blood stem from the more general perfusion deficit rather than from the ischemic heart alone. The blood lactate levels serve as an adequate prognosticator of survival. Increased blood lactate concentration with the accompanying acidosis may lead to potentially fatal arrhythmias.

Increased secretion of catecholamines, aldosterone and glucocorticoid is a more general feature of shock. The secretion of cortisol, and most probably aldosterone, is tripled.

Hyperglycemia, frequently observed in the presence of shock, is believed due to increased mobilization of glycogen, via increased catecholamine secretion, and anaerobic metabolism.

The usual metabolic behavior of the heart is changed following acute myocardial infarction. Whereas the normal heart metabolizes lactate, myocardial usage of lactate is decreased in experimental myocardial infarction, and oxygen extraction from the available blood supply is also reduced.

PULMONARY FUNCTION IN CARDIOGENIC SHOCK

Changes in pulmonary function are not yet completely understood. Some of the changes that have been determined are as follows:

1. The partial pressure of oxygen is reduced, even when patients are ventilated with 100% oxygen.
2. Effectively, large pulmonary arteriovenous shunts are established causing ventilation–perfusion inequities, the mechanism being unknown.
3. Major portions of the lung are underperfused. Consequently, the physiologic dead space is enlarged.
4. The defect in oxygen exchange is not due to failure of ventilation.

Irreversible Cardiogenic Shock[132]

As the complication of cardiogenic shock progresses to a more serious stage, certain physiologic changes become more dominant. The following are the processes by which the changes of irreversible shock occur (see Table 3).

1. The increased outpouring of corticosteroids and epinephrine and the increased sympathetic activity liberating increased amounts of norepinephrine at the neural junctions cause stimulation of receptors in effector organs.
2. The stimulation of the alpha receptors affects the peripheral circulation in the viscera and skin, and to a lesser extent in the muscle masses, and causes an intense vasoconstrictor effect on precapillary arteriolar sphincters as well as on postcapillary venular sphincters.

TABLE 3.—SCHEMATIC REPRESENTATION OF CARDIOGENIC SHOCK

1. Decreased myocardial contraction
   (via interruption of muscle continuity)
   ↓

2. Decreased cardiac output
   (ineffective "power" for pumping)
   ↓

3. Decreased aortic and carotid arterial pressure
   ↓

4. Activation of baroreceptors in aorta and carotid arteries
   ↓

5. Stimulation of sympathetic nervous system
   ↓

6. Norepinephrine and epinephrine (catecholamine) release
   ↓

7. Increased peripheral arterial resistance   ──────────→   COMPENSATED SHOCK
   (selective sparing of coronary and cerebral arteries)   MAY OCCUR—
   ⊥

   ⌐ If cardiac output continues to be decreased or falls ⌐
   └ even further   ┘
                        ↓

8. Increased sympathetic activity occurs with increased
   norepinephrine and epinephrine release, along with
   cortisol and aldosterone release
   ↓

9. Constriction of precapillary arterioles and
   postcapillary venules   ──────────→   ISCHEMIC ANOXIA
   (includes renal glomerular capillaries causing oliguria)
   ⊥

   ⌐ If shock is prolonged and uncompensated ⌐
   └   ┘
                        ↓

10. Accumulation of metabolic products, occurrence   ────────→   IRREVERSIBLE SHOCK
    of lactic acidosis with decreased pH   BEGINNING—
    ↓

11. Same vessels become less responsive to catecholamine
    effects
    ↓

12. Decreased responsiveness in turn causes liberation of
    more catecholamines via sympathetic nervous system stimulation
    ↓

13. Arteriolar sphincters no longer able to maintain tone; ────→   STAGNANT ANOXIA
    venular sphincters able to maintain tone;   OCCURRING—
    therefore blood accumulates in the capillaries in
    increasing amounts
    ↓

14. Increasing anoxia and acidosis occurs in the capillary beds
    ↓

15. Blood entering congested stagnant capillary beds has
    difficulty leaving capillary beds.
    ↓

16. Hydrostatic pressure in congested capillaries is higher
    than colloid pressure and fluid leaves capillary microcirculation
    ↓

17. Significant decrease in plasma volume

↓

18. More severe ischemia occurs in capillary microcirculation; sludging and thrombosis occur

↓

19. Capillary walls lose their integrity and disrupt

↓

20. Whole blood diffuses into tissues

↓

21. Further decrease in blood volume occurs potentiating irreversible shock

↓

22. Further derangement of cardiac and metabolic functions occurs via increased congestion (decreased venous return; decreased cardiac output, decreased coronary flow, decreased blood pH and further decrease in cardiac efficiency)

↓

23. Cardiac function deteriorates and arrest or fibrillation supervenes

---

3. The result of this reaction is to preserve, at all costs, the blood flow to the brain and heart, as the cerebral and coronary circulation systems are little affected by the vasoconstrictive effects of catecholamines (epinephrine and norepinephrine).

4. Shock at this phase of *ischemic anoxia* is usually readily reversible.

5. If shock is prolonged, the situation in the tissues gradually changes from pale ischemic anoxia to congested *stagnant anoxia*. Now we are approaching *irreversible shock*.

6. As a result of the vasoconstriction in arterioles and venules, products of metabolism accumulate, leading to acidosis and a lowered pH. This situation in turn causes these same vessels to be less responsive to the effects of catecholamines.

7. The decreased responsiveness in turn results in increased norepinephrine liberation by the sympathetic nervous system and increased epinephrine secretion by the adrenal medulla.
   a. This response of the sympathetic nervous system occurs in order to maintain vasoconstriction in the face of increasing acidosis and therefore in the face of decreasing effectiveness of catecholamines.

8. Eventually, if shock is prolonged, the arteriolar sphincters are no longer able to maintain tone despite heroic attempts by the body to secrete additional vasoactive substances.

9. With the loss of arteriolar tone, blood can now get into the capillary beds in increasing amounts.

10. However, for some unexplained reason, the venular sphincters are still able to maintain reasonably normal tone in the face of severe acidosis of shock.
    a. This may be due to the fact that the venular sphincters normally function at a pH lower than those on the arterial side.

11. The result is that blood may enter the capillary beds but has difficulty in leaving these stagnant capillary beds.

12. Hydrostatic pressure within the congested capillaries increases above colloid osmotic pressure, and fluid begins to leave the microcirculation in increasing amounts, becoming extravascular fluid.
    a. Significant losses (30–40% of plasma volume) can be measured in dogs suffering shock from a variety of causes.

13. As this process of stagnation continues, ischemia may become so severe that the capillaries lose their integrity and slough, allowing whole blood to diffuse into the tissues.
    a. This diffusion further reduces the blood volume, increasing and potentiating irreversible shock.

14. The increasing congestion diminishes venous return.
    a. This in turn further lowers cardiac output and coronary flow.
    b. Moreover, the lowered blood pH further decreases cardiac efficiency.
    c. Eventually cardiac function deteriorates and arrest or fibrillation supervenes.

Therapy of Cardiogenic Shock

THE PRESENT

There are many pharmacologic methods of therapy for cardiogenic shock currently proposed in the literature. To further add to the confusion of determining which therapeutic regimen to use, essentially all the proposed methods are well substantiated by experimental and clinical investigation. For our purposes we will present a listing of the pharmacologic agents used, a sampling of the regimens employed and a suggested routine for therapy.

Further understanding of underlying pharmacophysiology may be derived by reviewing Chapter 15.

The rather classic method of therapy for cardiogenic shock utilizing the sympathomimetic amines norepinephrine (Levophed) or metaraminol (Aramine) is the most used therapy for cardiogenic shock at present. However, extremely valid arguments for other regimens and good results from their use have been presented.

CURRENT GENERAL METHODS

A gross presentation of the methods of therapy currently utilized in association with therapy of cardiogenic shock is as follows:

1. Agents which are both alpha and beta adrenergic stimulating (norepinephrine and metaraminol).
2. Alpha and beta adrenergic stimulating agents in conjunction with alpha-blocking agents (norepinephrine and alpha blockage with phentolamine; or alpha blockage with pharmacologic doses of glucocorticosteroids, phenoxybenzamine or chlorpromazine).
3. Beta adrenergic stimulating agents with or without intravascular volume-expanding agents (e.g., isoproterenol with or without low molecular weight dextran or whole blood).

THE FUTURE

It is probable that in time a careful subdivision of patients with acute myocardial infarction and cardiogenic shock will be made. This subdivision will necessarily be one of hemodynamic groups. It may be possible in the future to define precisely those individuals who will respond in a predictable and beneficial manner to one of the various methods of therapy. This will undoubtedly require rapid, on-line, computerized determinations of hemodynamic and metabolic alterations and will also require previously determined, known responses to various pharmacologic and physical agents utilized in specific subdivisions of hemodynamic groups. Further investigation, with detailed measurement of sequential hemodynamic, metabolic and clinical effects, will be required before this is possible.

Pharmacologic Agents and Their Dosages*

LEVARTERENOL (NOREPINEPHRINE, LEVOPHED)

1. IV 4–8 mg. in 1,000 ml. 5% D/W or D/S by infusion.
2. Both an alpha and a beta adrenergic stimulator, with predominantly alpha stimulation. It increases peripheral resistance and cardiac output.

*References: 1, 7, 14, 25.

a. Blood pressure is brought to 90–100 mm. Hg systolic. Higher pressures may produce reflex bradycardia and decrease cardiac output.
b. Level of blood pressure desired depends on blood pressure before onset of cardiogenic shock.
c. If extravasation occurs, there may be tissue sloughing. Try to place infusion in upper extremity.
   1) If extravasation occurs, infiltrate area with phentolamine (Regitine), 3–5 ml. diluted in 10–30 ml. saline (depending on the size of the ischemic area).
3. See Chapter 15.

METARAMINOL (ARAMINE)[136]

1. IV, 25–100 mg. in 500–1,000 ml. 5% D/W. Drip at rate of 10–30 drops/minute until systolic blood pressure is 90–100.
2. See Chapter 15.

ISOPROTERENOL (ISUPREL)[10,25,98,131,136,140,160,183]

1. IV, 1 mg. in 500 ml. 5% D/W (2 μg./ml.). Start at 10 drops/minute.
a. Infusion rates of 0.5 μg./minute have been recommended.
b. At doses of 2 μg./minute, isoproterenol was found not to induce ectopic ventricular activity.[160] At doses greater than 6 μg./minute, ectopic ventricular activity does occur at times.
c. When volume of fluid infusion is important, concentrations up to 10 times greater have been used. Adjust the drip rate accordingly.
d. Speed of infusion adjusted on the basis of heart rate, central venous pressure, systemic blood pressure and urine flow.
   1) Heart rates exceeding 110 beats/minute: It may be advisable to decrease the infusion rate.
   2) Doses of isoproterenol sufficient to increase the heart rate to more than 120–130 beats/minute may induce ventricular arrhythmias.[10,25]
2. See Chapter 15.

DIGITALIS

Cardiac glycosides are frequently used in the presence of cardiogenic shock. Indications for use are given here.

1. Digitalis is an excellent inotropic agent, does not increase oxygen demand and, when properly used, may possibly have less potential for cardiac arrhythmias than sympathomimetic amines (including Isuprel).
2. A prime indication for digitalization is elevated central venous pressure. Overt clinical failure in cardiogenic shock is a definite indication. Digitalization in cardiogenic shock should be carried out intravenously.

3. The rationale for early digitalization in cardiogenic shock is that it may prove helpful in individual situations because:
   a. Heart failure frequently accompanies shock.
   b. Digitalis has positive inotropic effect.
   c. There are resultant reflex peripheral effects of digitalization.
   d. Some authorities feel all patients suffering from cardiogenic shock who are over age 50 should be digitalized.[132]
   e. *Note:* Proper assessment of serum potassium levels must be done.

DEXTRAN (LOW MOLECULAR WEIGHT)

1. When cardiogenic shock is being treated by agents which lower the peripheral resistance, the resultant hypovolemia must be treated by a suitable volume expansion agent. If the hematocrit value is adequate, the agent of choice is probably low molecular weight (40,000 average) dextran.
2. The clinical indication for low molecular weight dextran is determined entirely by the central venous pressure, which must be monitored if the agent is given. Dextran should not be given to patients with high central venous pressures because pulmonary edema may be precipitated.[179] Dextran also has other beneficial effects on the microcirculation (see Chapter 16).
   a. Dextran is preferred because:
      1) Dextran 40 has an osmotic, diuretic effect on kidneys.
      2) Hypertonicity of dextran 40 attracts volume from extravascular space almost equal to that volume administered.

STEROIDS

1. Glucocorticosteroids are utilized in pharmacologic doses (not physiologic doses) in the treatment of cardiogenic shock. The purpose of steroids in cardiogenic shock is predominantly to decrease peripheral resistance; however, other beneficial effects may accrue. (See Steroids in Chapter 16.)
2. Dosage Schedules.
   a. Hydrocortisone sodium succinate (Solu-Cortef), 150 mg./kg. IV over a period of a few minutes.[134]
      1) Acts in 5 minutes.
      2) Maximal effects occur in 1½-2 hours.
      3) Repeat in 1-2 hours[123,132,150] or 4-6 hours.[124]
      4) Pharmacologic, *not* physiologic dose. Gradually decreases peripheral resistance, expanding size of vascular space.
      5) Hydrocortisone IV in doses of 50 mg./kg. acts as an alpha adrenergic blocking agent.[123,132]
      6) Give steroid only if central venous pressure is over 10 cm. water.

   a) If central venous pressure is lower, volume replacement with low molecular weight dextran, blood or plasma is carried out.
      (1) The choice of volume expander depends on hematocrit determination.
      (2) Dextran is preferred if hematocrit is normal.
   7) If shock continues over 4 hours, look for other contributing causes.
   b. Dosage schedules for analogs of cortisone.
      1) Prednisolone (succinate or phosphate), 250 mg. IV. Repeat in 4-6 hours.[124]
      2) Methyl prednisolone (succinate), 250 mg. IV. Repeat in 4-6 hours.[124] Or 30 mg./kg. IV bolus.[134]
      3) Dexamethasone (phosphate), 20 mg. IV. Repeat in 6-8 hours.[124] Or 6 mg./kg. IV bolus.[134]
3. Pharmacologic consideration of cortisone analogs. The major determinant of the concentration of cortisol or cortisol derivative at the receptor site is the resistance of the corticosteroid molecule to metabolic alteration. For this reason analogs of cortisol (prednisolone, 6-methyl-prednisolone, triamcinolone and dexamethasone) may be preferable; they equilibrate more rapidly between blood and tissues since they do not compete with cortisol for its plasma protein-binding sites,[124] and thus do not undergo metabolic alteration as rapidly.
4. Features of therapy. The important features of corticosteroid therapy in the treatment of shock are:
   a. The therapy must be prompt.
   b. Very high—pharmacologic—doses must be used.
   c. The duration of therapy must be of the shortest possible time.[124]

PHENOXYBENZAMINE (POB, DIBENZYLINE)

1. POB is an alpha adrenergic blocking agent. A hazard of the drug is that it decreases peripheral vascular resistance and should not be used unless central venous pressure is monitored. This drug does not yet have approval of the Food and Drug Administration for this type of use and must be considered experimental.
2. The usual IV dose is 1 mg./kg. diluted in 100 ml. 5% D/W and infused over 2-4 hours.[130,135]
   a. This drug acts within minutes to decrease peripheral resistance.
   b. Central venous pressure is maintained at 10-12 cm. water before, during and for 24 hours after the drug is given via volume expanders.
   c. The choice of volume expander depends on the hematocrit value.[135]
      1) With a normal hematocrit, give either plasma or low molecular weight dextran. (Dextran has advantages—see Chapter 16.)
3. See Chapter 15.

PHENTOLAMINE (REGITINE)

1. This alpha adrenergic blocking agent has been used in conjunction with norepinephrine (combined norepinephrine and phentolamine) in the treatment of shock. Some investigators have found that the combination[181] is more effective than norepinephrine alone.
   a. 5 mg. Regitine is added to a 1,000 ml. D/W 5% mixture of norepinephrine (1 ml. Regitine ampule contains 5 mg.).
2. The above therapy combines an alpha and beta stimulator and an alpha-blocking agent.
3. Phentolamine (Regitine) has numerous side effects, other than its alpha adrenergic blockade effect, which makes it unsatisfactory in large doses.

CHLORPROMAZINE (THORAZINE)

1. Mechanism of action: Both chlorpromazine and phenoxybenzamine act by blocking the effects of catecholamines on the alpha receptors of the pre- and postcapillary arterioles and venules of the skin and viscera. These receptors have not been located anatomically, but their presence has been functionally demonstrated pharmacologically. Chlorpromazine thus acts as an alpha adrenergic blocking agent.
2. Usually given IV in a dose of 1 mg./kg., chlorpromazine should be given over a 10–15 minute period.[135]
   a. Central venous pressure must be monitored as for phenoxybenzamine.
   b. Chlorpromazine does not produce the dramatic increases in vascular capacitance seen with phenoxybenzamine because its alpha-blocking effects are not nearly as strong.
   c. A volume expander must be used to maintain central venous pressure, just as with phenoxybenzamine.
3. *Caution:* The hazard of these and similar-acting drugs is the dramatic increase in vascular capacity that results from their use. These drugs should therefore NOT be used unless the physician is willing to monitor the central venous pressure during and after their administration.[135]

3-HYDROXYTYRAMINE (DOPAMINE)

1. Dopamine (3-hydroxytyramine) has had limited clinical investigation, and should be considered experimental at present. This drug has been studied in cardiogenic shock in both animals and man.[168,180]
2. Dopamine is a precursor of norepinephrine in the metabolic formation of that chemical adrenergic neurotransmitter, having both beta stimulating and selective alpha receptor effects (apparently both alpha stimulation and blockade).
3. The dosage used in several patients has ranged from 0.5 to 10.0 μg./kg./minute.
   a. Therapy has been initiated with a small dose of 0.5 μg./kg./minute which would seem to be prudent until more study with the drug leads to the development of a more specific protocol.
   b. ECG monitoring should be carried out during administration.
4. See Chapter 15.

Methods of Therapy

As previously mentioned, there are many regimens for the therapy of cardiogenic shock. Several will be presented here as examples, and a specific suggested routine presented. At a future time, some combination of these methods or some totally new methods may prove to be most effective. It may also be that, at present, one method may be more satisfactory for milder cardiogenic shock, with lesser decreases in cardiac output, and another method may be more satisfactory for more severe shock, with greater decreases in cardiac output. This possibility exists even in the same patient in varying degrees of cardiogenic shock.

GUIDELINES FOR THERAPY[14,42,98,158,179]

Certain measurements, guidelines and general therapeutic measures are either essential or desirable in all methods of therapy for cardiogenic shock. These will be outlined before a description of the various methods of therapy.

1. **Oxygen.** Deliver a high concentration of oxygen by face mask or nasal cannula.
2. **Monitor physiologic data.** Monitoring the following physiologic data is desirable, when possible:
   a. Blood pressure.
   b. Cardiac output.
   c. Peripheral arterial resistance.
   d. Heart rate.
   e. Central venous pressure.
   f. Circulation time.
3. **Monitor urine flow.** The rate of urine flow is an excellent guide to the effect of all agents in the therapy of cardiogenic shock.
   a. If therapy is effective, urine flow should be in excess of 0.5 ml./minute.
      1) An indwelling catheter is necessary to determine accurately the rate of urine flow from the kidneys.
   b. Measure fluid intake and output carefully.
      1) Record the urine volume and commence monitoring urinary output from the time of initiating therapy.
4. **Other gross indicators.** Warmth of the extremities and volume of the pulse are also excellent gross indicators of the patient's response to therapy.
5. **Blood pressure.** Arterial pressure must be carefully monitored.

a. Arterial blood pressure alone may be misleading as a guide to regulation of cardiogenic shock therapy. It is possible to have hypotension without shock.

b. Careful clinical observation must be made of the other signs and symptoms of shock, and their correction must be undertaken.

c. Do not raise the blood pressure too high with vasopressors.
   1) There is evidence that raising the systolic blood pressure above approximately 90 mm. Hg in a previously normotensive individual is associated with decreased cardiac output.
   2) Try to ascertain the pretreatment blood pressure level. In previously hypertensive patients the "best" blood pressure level obtainable with vasopressor drugs is not satisfactorily known.
   3) Do not be discouraged by a zero blood pressure reading on the blood pressure cuff.
      a) Often intra-arterial pressure determinations may indicate 10–30 mm. Hg in this situation.

d. Do not be content with satisfactory vasopressor effect alone. Other changes in cardiogenic shock must be corrected. If increasing oliguria or coma occurs despite adequate blood pressure cuff readings, the clinical condition of the patient is deteriorating.

e. Do not discontinue pressor drugs or monitoring after only a short time of hemodynamic stability (e.g., 15–30 minutes, when 1–3 hours is preferable). The length of time must be determined individually.

6. **Monitor central venous pressure.** Use central venous pressure determinations, if possible, because they:
   a. Are more reliable than peripheral venous pressure measurements.
   b. Are an excellent guide to safe volume replacement during fluid disturbance.
      1) Indicate the ability of the heart to receive blood returned to it and to eject the blood.
   c. Aid in differentiating congestive heart failure from shock.
      1) An initial reading of 20 cm. water is usually caused by congestive heart failure.
   d. The central venous catheter may be used to accomplish phlebotomy, if that becomes necessary.
      1) It facilitates withdrawal of blood for electrolyte or biochemical measurements.

7. **Electrolyte and biochemical measurements.**
   a. Measure blood lactate if possible.
      1) This determination reflects to some degree the severity of the shock state; and the acidosis, reflected by this finding, may itself lead to death.
   b. Obtain pH determinations, if possible. Blood from the central venous catheter may be used.
      1) Acidosis and alkalosis may interfere with

pressor drug response. There may be metabolic inhibition of the ability of the peripheral vessels to respond to vasopressors in the presence of marked acidosis or anoxia.
      2) These patients may respond to measures to correct acidosis in association with measures to improve blood flow in the microcirculation.

8. **IV Catheter.** For infusing vasopressor solutions use a plastic intravenous catheter rather than an ordinary intravenous needle. The catheter is preferably inserted into a vein in the upper extremity to decrease the danger of sloughing if extravasation occurs. Polyethylene and Teflon catheter apparatus are available.

SIMULTANEOUS CARDIOGENIC SHOCK AND PULMONARY EDEMA

Clinically, cardiogenic shock and heart failure (manifested by pulmonary edema or congestive heart failure) may coexist.

1. Pulmonary edema may develop as a late complication of shock, or vice versa.
2. The combination occurs frequently and poses a serious therapeutic problem.
3. Treat cardiogenic shock and pulmonary edema simultaneously, as follows:
   a. Treat shock as per usual method.
   b. Minimize IV fluids.
      1) Use glucose instead of sodium chloride.
   c. Other than vasopressors, use all measures considered to combat pulmonary edema.
      1) Place patient in the sitting position only if blood pressure is adequately corrected.
      2) Aminophylline is administered only if blood pressure is well controlled, due to the drug's hypotensive effect.
      3) Phlebotomy is contraindicated in severe shock.
   d. IV digitalization is required.

SPECIFIC METHODS OF THERAPY

Method I (Alpha and beta stimulating drugs)

1. Administration of norepinephrine (Levophed).[1,25,179]
   a. IV infusion, 4–8 mg. base in 1,000 ml. 5% D/W. Infuse until blood pressure is approximately 90 mm. Hg systolic, and observe for change in other signs of shock.
   b. Norepinephrine increases cardiac output in 90% of patients with cardiogenic shock.[179]
   c. With patients not responding to norepinephrine, administration of sodium bicarbonate may restore peripheral vascular responsiveness.
      1) Serum pH and lactic acid determinations may help determine acidosis.

2. Metaraminol (Aramine)
   a. A norepinephrine-releasing drug.
   b. 100 mg. in 1,000 5% D/W by infusion until there is appropriate blood pressure response.

Method II (Alpha and beta stimulation with alpha blockade)

1. Norepinephrine (Levophed), 4–8 mg. in 1,000 ml. 5% D/W.
2. In addition, administer one of the alpha adrenergic blocking drugs, as follows:
   a. Phentolamine (Regitine), 5 mg. into the same 1,000-ml. bottle of fluid containing the norepinephrine.[181]
   b. Phenoxybenzamine (Dibenzyline) 1 mg./kg. IV.[132]
   c. Glucocorticosteroid in pharmacologic doses[132,133] (see p. 47).
   d. Chlorpromazine (Thorazine) IV[133] (see p. 48).
3. Additional considerations using this method of therapy.
   a. Digitalization is usually carried out.[130]
   b. Volume expanders are administered as needed, use of whole blood, plasma or dextran depending on the hematocrit value.[132]
      1) A central venous catheter is placed for central venous pressure monitoring.
      2) With a normal hematocrit, dextran is most beneficial. (See Chapter 16.)

Method III (Beta adrenergic stimulation with or without volume expansion)

1. Isoproterenol (Isuprel) IV, 1 mg. in 500 ml. 5% D/W. Start infusion at 10 drops/minute. (See Isoproterenol, p. 46 and Chapter 9.)
   a. Digitalis may be used in conjunction. Watch for digitalis toxicity.
   b. Some acute coronary care units use this method exclusively.[140]
   c. In some studies, isoproterenol has been found superior to norepinephrine in experimental shock [75,98] and superior to metaraminol in man. [136] In some studies it has been found to be inferior to norepinephrine.[183]
   d. Lidocaine has been administered concomitantly to overcome the myocardial irritant effects of isoproterenol.[75]
2. Volume expansion is frequently utilized. The volume expanders used are whole blood, plasma or dextran, and the choice is dependent on the hematocrit reading.
   a. Low hematocrit, use whole blood.
   b. High hematocrit, use plasma or dextran.
   c. Dextran has been studied in experimental shock in conjunction with isoproterenol and lidocaine and found to be beneficial.[75]

3. This method of therapy might be desirable for severe or so-called irreversible cardiogenic shock.

The Future

All pharmacologic methods of treatment leave much to be desired. The role of mechanical aids, particularly intra-aortic balloon mechanisms, will probably increase.[261]

More adequate classification of the degrees of cardiogenic shock for therapeutic purposes will probably also be forthcoming.

Suggested Routine for Therapy

(For further information on individual drugs and drug dosages, see Pharmacologic Agents and Their Dosages, this chapter, and Drugs Affecting the Autonomic Nervous System, Chapter 15.)

It is impossible to present an inflexible guide for the treatment of cardiogenic shock, since each patient must be treated individually on the basis of clinical assessment. The following is an attempt to present a general guideline for therapy of cardiogenic shock.

MILD DEGREES OF SHOCK

1. The patient with a mild degree of shock has the following manifestations:
   a. Mild to moderate hypotension (systolic pressure of 70–90 mm. Hg).
   b. Minimum signs and symptoms of the low perfusion syndrome (mild sweating, cool but not cold skin, euphoria, mildly elevated pulse rate).
   c. Adequate but decreased urinary output—if close measurements have been done.
2. For the patient with a mild degree of shock the following routine is suggested:
   a. Norepinephrine (Levophed), 4–8 mg. base in 1,000 ml. of 5% D/W at a rate sufficient to maintain blood pressure at about 90 mm. Hg systolic, with clearing signs and symptoms of shock.
   b. Early digitalization may be desirable.
   c. Insert a Foley catheter.

MORE SEVERE SHOCK

1. More aggressive therapy must be initiated if any of the following occur:
   a. Blood pressure, signs and symptoms do not respond to the above therapy in 15–30 minutes.
   b. Urinary output decreases below 0.5 ml./minute early in therapy or later in therapy.
   c. Clinical condition deteriorates after a period of successful therapy, and particularly if there is not

adequate response to an increased rate of nore-pinephrine (Levophed) drip.
2. The following basic routine is suggested:
   a. Continue Levophed or increase the rate of IV drip, and/or change concentration to 16 mg. Levophed base per 1,000 ml. D/5/W.
   b. Give Dexamethasone (Decadron, Hexadrol), 20 mg. IV (pharmacologic dose). Repeat in 1½–4 hours.
   c. Insert central venous pressure catheter and monitor central venous pressure (CVP).
   d. Administer a volume expander, if necessary: this is determined by CVP reading or changes.
      1) Dextran 40 is given if the hematocrit is normal. Blood may be necessary if the hematocrit is low.
   e. Digitalize via the IV route, if this was not previously done.
   f. Correct acidosis. Measure electrolytes, lactic acid, pH.
   g. Carefully measure urine output; the output should be greater than 0.5 ml./minute.

SEVERE SHOCK—SUSPECTED IRREVERSIBLE SHOCK

If the therapy for More Severe Shock is not effective after 30–45 minutes, as judged by the criteria set forth for initiating that therapy, the following routine is suggested:
1. Isoproterenol (Isuprel), 1 mg. in 500 ml. D/5/W, is substituted for the Levophed.
   a. Lidocaine (Xylocaine) drip—as for treatment of VPCs—may be used simultaneously to control the myocardial irritant effects of Isuprel.
2. Volume expansion is used as needed.
3. Follow other methods of therapy as outlined under More Severe Shock.

CHAPTER 6

Other Immediate Life-threatening Complications

Congestive Heart Failure

Definition

Congestive heart failure (CHF) is one of the manifestations of backward failure, in which the body fails to eliminate fluid. With the occurrence of CHF, the central venous pressure increases and congestion of the organs occurs. Along with an accumulation of fluid, there is sodium and water retention, mediated by kidney and adrenal responses.

Variable Degrees

Congestive failure occurs in varying degrees, depending on the stage of progression of the process, and may be mild, moderate, severe or acute pulmonary edema. (Acute pulmonary edema is a part of the total spectrum of CHF.)

Heart failure seen in acute myocardial infarction is usually the rapidly developing type and is usually referred to as *left ventricular failure* in cardiac literature.

Congestive heart failure is usually manifested by distended peripheral veins, peripheral edema, basilar rales, possibly hepatomegaly, increased pulse rate, dyspnea and increased weight. These changes occur secondary to increased filling pressure of the right atrium. The increased right atrial pressure can be measured by measuring central venous pressure.

Therapy

Digitalization is the primary therapy, increasing the inotropy of the heart and reducing the right atrial filling pressure. Other treatment may necessitate some portion of that treatment recommended for pulmonary edema, depending on the speed of onset and severity of the congestive failure. Diet low in sodium, occasionally fluid restriction and various dosages of one of the diuretics are also utilized. Elastic stockings or wrap should be used to aid in the prevention of thromboembolic phenomena. If at all possible, anticoagulation measures should also be carried out in the presence of acute myocardial infarction. Mechanical removal of fluid (pleural effusion or ascites) may be necessary if fluid accumulates in the body cavities.

Discussion

Congestive heart failure is frequently seen as a manifestation of arteriosclerotic heart disease. However, with acute myocardial infarction the slow onset type of CHF classically seen with arteriosclerotic heart disease is seldom observed. The slower onset type of CHF is seldom seen in the coronary care unit due to the relatively short stay of the patient in the unit. Mechanical or "power" heart failure most usually seen in the coronary care unit commonly has a relatively rapid onset, most frequently developing in a few hours to a few days. This rapid onset type of CHF is usually predominantly a manifestation of the acute heart muscle injury and the markedly decreased myocardial contraction that accompanies this injury. The classic slow onset type customarily seen outside the coronary care unit is also initiated by "power" failure of the myocardium, but the mechanical failure is usually of gradual onset, and hemodynamic abnormalities develop much more slowly in this situation than in the presence of acute myocardial injury.

Congestive heart failure of the rapid onset type is treated in essentially the same manner as the classic slower onset CHF seen with arteriosclerotic heart disease in the absence of acute myocardial infarction. For this reason little space is devoted here to the pathologic physiology or therapy of congestive heart failure, as there are numerous excellent reference sources available for this study.

It should be noted, however, that the *tempo of therapy* of CHF accompanying acute myocardial infarction may necessarily be *faster* than that in the classic more slowly developing type.

Pulmonary Edema

INTRODUCTION

Pulmonary edema is a manifestation of left-sided heart failure whereby, due to mechanical inefficiency, the left side of the heart cannot maintain an adequate output of the venous blood brought to the left ventricle from the pulmonary circulation. Pure left-sided failure may occur with acute myocardial infarction. Pulmonary edema represents the very rapid onset of CHF and as such is a manifestation of the total symptom spectrum of CHF.

Personnel caring for the acute coronary patient must anticipate the possibility of some degree of heart failure accompanying acute myocardial infarction. The presence of basilar or dependent rales, detected early after acute myocardial infarction, will usually indicate that the patient should be treated with digitalis. The presence of dependent rales will indicate that interstitial edema has occurred and alveolar edema is occurring.

If acute pulmonary edema suddenly appears, either as paroxysmal nocturnal dyspnea (PND) or as full-blown clinical pulmonary edema, it will demand immediate and active therapy to prevent death due to this manifestation of mechanical ("power") failure. Unfortunately the availability of the acute coronary care unit and continuous ECG monitoring has had little effect on the mortality due to this type of mechanical heart failure.

When changes of pulmonary edema have progressed to an advanced degree, or if this major complication does not respond to vigorous therapy, the resultant anoxia and attendant electrolyte disturbances often produce secondary arrhythmias as a terminal event.

PATHOLOGIC PHYSIOLOGY—PROGRESSIVE STAGES AND SYMPTOMS

1. Pulmonary edema is a manifestation of left-sided heart failure in which the heart is unable to pump adequately into the systemic circulation the venous blood returning to the left heart from the pulmonary circulation. *Pulmonary venous hypertension* is the first stage in the process of pulmonary edema. There is a rise in pulmonary capillary pressure, which must reach 25–30 mm. Hg before pulmonary edema occurs.[165]

2. After the occurrence of increased capillary pressure there is a transudation of fluid into the interstitial spaces *between* the alveoli of the lungs. This is a manifestation of the retrograde transmission of the increased pressure in the pulmonary system and is referred to as *interstitial edema* (also sometimes referred to as pulmonary congestion).

   a. At this stage in the pathologic process of pulmonary edema the clinical manifestations include nothing more than slight dyspnea.

   b. It has been shown that a large undetected percentage of patients with acute myocardial infarction progress to this stage of pulmonary congestion, demonstrated on chest films as a feathery appearance in the perihilar area.[125,221] Rales cannot be heard in the lungs. Chest films taken at this stage for any reason might reveal the changes. Some clinicians begin digitalis therapy at this time if no contraindications are present.

3. If acute pulmonary hypertension persists and increases, the next stage of development is the transudation of fluid into the alveolar spaces. Pulmonary edema becomes clinically manifest if alveolar fluid is present in sufficient degree. The clinical manifestations are increasing dyspnea and cough. The patient will have noticeable dyspnea and cough as this stage occurs and progresses, and rales are heard in the dependent portions of the lungs.

   Often improvement in symptoms will occur if the patient is placed in the sitting position, thus allowing lung volume and vital capacity of the lungs to increase, along with a decrease in venous blood return to the heart. The improvement is caused by a relative pooling of the blood below the level of the heart.

   a. Paroxysmal nocturnal dyspnea (PND).
      With the patient in the recumbent position, sudden decompensation of the left heart may begin, causing the alveoli to fill with large amounts of fluid. Marked dyspnea, cough and cyanosis follow. These signs actually herald the onset of acute pulmonary edema, and the condition derives its name from the fact that it usually occurs at night (nocturnal) while the patient is recumbent, is sudden in onset (thus making it paroxysmal), and the patient is markedly dyspneic. This situation demands the same vigorous therapy as other manifestations of pulmonary edema.

4. The subsequent stage of the pathologic process is full-blown pulmonary edema. The patient's coughing increases and he becomes cyanotic; there are rasping sounds from the respiratory tree; the pulse rate increases; the patient perspires profusely, though the skin is cool (even in the absence of shock); the cough then becomes incessant; frothy sputum is present, frequently coming out the mouth; the sputum then becomes both bloody and frothy; and there can be no doubt that the diagnosis is pulmonary edema.

   Mild to moderate dyspnea may develop into full-blown pulmonary edema in a very short time.

VARIABLE FACTORS AFFECTING THERAPY

The treatment of acute pulmonary hypertension

and pulmonary congestion or edema varies according to the following factors:

1. Stage of progression of the pathologic process.
2. Speed of progression of the pathologic process.
3. Previous therapy and the time elapsed since that therapy was received. Assessment of the last therapy with digitalis, diuretics, sedation and antiarrhythmic drugs is particularly important.
4. Presence or absence of other major complications of acute myocardial infarction, particularly previously treated congestive heart failure, cardiogenic shock and arrhythmias.

OBJECTIVES OF THERAPY

The several objectives of therapy of pulmonary edema are outlined as follows:

1. Physical and mental relaxation.
   a. Decrease the physical work of tense muscles.
   b. Decrease the increased respiration of anxiety.
2. Relieve hypoxia.
3. Improve cardiovascular function.
   a. Strengthen the contractility of the heart muscle, thereby providing more efficient mechanical pumping effect.
4. Retard the return of venous blood to the heart.
   a. Retard the return of venous blood from the periphery of the body (extremities and lower portion of the body).
   b. Retard the return of venous blood from the pulmonary circulation.
   c. Decrease venous return and venous pressure by decreasing circulating fluid volume.

THERAPEUTIC MEASURES

Depending on the variable factors affecting the pathologic process of pulmonary edema, the objectives of therapy are achieved by one or more of the following therapeutic measures. After each of the therapeutic measures listed below will be found numerical references to the Objectives of Therapy (listed just previously) achieved by that particular measure.

1. Place patient in sitting (or Fowler's position (2, 4a).
   a. Increases lung volume and vital capacity, thus helps anoxia.
2. Morphine sulfate (1, 4a).
   a. May be given IV slowly, 8–15 mg. used.
   b. Sedates patient and decreases musculoskeletal and respiratory activity.
   c. Produces venous pooling, thus in effect performing a medical phlebotomy.
   d. Observe carefully for depressed ventilation in the face of an already hypoxic respiratory system.
      1) Have respiratory assistance available.
      2) Antagonist is Nalline (nalorphine).
      3) Contraindicated in the previously asthmatic patient.
3. Start oxygen by nasal catheter or cannula, if not already started (2).

a. Preferably 100% oxygen. High flow rates are necessary.
   1) Oxygen should be warm and saturated with water vapor.
4. Apply rotating tourniquets (bloodless phlebotomy) (4c).
   a. See protocol in Appendix for rotating tourniquets procedure.
   b. Maintain tourniquets with sufficient force to be greater than venous but less than arterial pressure. Apply to 3 extremities only and rotate every 15 minutes. At conclusion take tourniquets off one extremity at a time—to prevent sudden vascular overload.
5. Digitalis IV, in a rapid-acting preparation, if not already given (3a).
6. Aminophyllin IV (2, 3a, 4c).
   a. Give 240–480 mg. at a rate of 20–40 mg./minute.
   b. Inject drug slowly; side effects of headache, palpitation, dizziness, nausea, hypotension and cardiac arrhythmias may occur if injected rapidly IV.
   c. Acts as mild diuretic, relieves bronchospasm occurring in acute pulmonary edema, has cardiotonic effect and lowers venous pressure by relaxing smooth muscles of blood vessels. (N.B.: Relaxant effect on the smooth muscle of blood vessels can cause hypotension.)
   d. Use with caution in the presence of low blood pressure.
7. Diuretics (3, 4c).
   a. Mercuhydrin or Thiomerin IM. This is a holdover from treatment prior to the availability of strong, rapid-acting IM and IV diuretics.
   b. Furosemide (Lasix), 20 mg. IM, begins acting fairly rapidly, though not as rapidly as the same diuretic IV (see Diuretics, Chapter 13).
      1) Furosemide, 20–120 mg. IV, begins acting in minutes, peak action in 30–60 minutes.
   c. Ethacrynic acid (Edecrin), 50 mg. IV, rapid acting, with peak action in 30–60 minutes (See Diuretics, Chapter 13).
      1) May be given orally, 50–200 mg.
   d. IV diuretics given in excess will cause a profound diuresis, with water and electrolyte depletion. Administration may be lifesaving, but the patient should be observed for electrolyte imbalance following use, particularly the serum potassium and chloride levels. The levels of blood urea nitrogen and uric acid may also be raised. These changes are particularly important in those patients receiving digitalis.
8. Intermittent Positive Pressure Breathing (IPPB) (2, 4b).
   a. Effective but temporary measure. Literally dams up the pulmonary alveolar fluid. If the basic defects are not corrected, IPPB alone will not suffice.
   b. Deliver 100% oxygen via well-fitting mask.

c. Use defoaming agent. Ethyl alcohol is usually used in 30, 50 or 95% strength.[71] Synthetic 2-ethylhexanol has been used as a defoaming agent.[71]

d. Avoid high settings, as excess pressure decreases peripheral venous return and can cause an increase in circulatory collapse via *not enough* blood to the left heart and decreased left heart output. (Use 4–9 cm. water, low pressure setting.)

9. Phlebotomy of 300–500 ml. (4a, c).
   a. Phlebotomy is very effective therapy and the fastest way of reducing return of blood to the heart.
   b. If circulatory collapse is present, care is indicated since phlebotomy will aggravate shock.

10. Vasopressors. (See also Simultaneous Cardiogenic Shock and Pulmonary Edema in Chapter 5.)
    a. If cardiogenic shock develops, do the following:
       1) IV infusion of Levophed (norepinephrine), metaraminol (Aramine) or isoproterenol (Isuprel).
       2) Stop IPPB.
       3) Release tourniquets; no phlebotomy.

11. Antibiotics. Some clinicians use "prophylactic" antibiotics when pulmonary edema or pulmonary congestion is present. There is no definite evidence that this practice reduces the incidence of pneumonia and it may result in formation of resistant organisms.

Rupture of the Myocardium

SITES OF RUPTURE

The myocardium may rupture in the event of acute myocardial infarction at any of 3 sites. These are the ventricle, the intraventricular septum and the papillary muscle. Each of these will be considered separately.

RUPTURE OF THE VENTRICLE (RUPTURE OF THE HEART)

1. Incidence and Prognosis

Rupture of the ventricle is said to account for 5–7% of the sudden deaths that occur during the first week after acute myocardial infarction. Rupture of the ventricle nearly always occurs within the first 2 weeks following infarct.[71]

Death following ventricular rupture is inevitable and usually within minutes. Death occurs via hemopericardium and cardiac tamponade.

2. Pathologic Physiology

a. Usually extensive transmural damage is necessary in order for ventricular rupture to occur.
b. For massive transmural infarction to develop, there is nearly always extensive disease of more than one major coronary artery, depriving the injured area of its primary blood supply and its sources of collateral circulation simultaneously.[13]
   1) Sudden acute occlusion of a single coronary artery rarely may lead to ventricular rupture.
c. The laceration in the myocardium which leads to rupture does not occur as a sharply defined localized blowout, but as an irregular dissection of the ventricular wall.[71]
d. Rupture occurs more commonly through the anterior surface of the left ventricle.
e. Whether excessive early ambulation contributes to weakening of the healing process is disputed at present.[13,71]
f. Whether the use of anticoagulants is a contributing cause is undetermined, but is thought not to be a usual factor.

RUPTURE OF THE INTRAVENTRICULAR SEPTUM

1. Incidence and Prognosis

a. Rupture of intraventricular septum is said to account for 2% of all deaths following acute myocardial infarction.[71]
b. The prognosis of intraventricular septal rupture is extremely poor. Most patients with ruptured intraventricular septum die within the first week after infarct.
c. Rupture of the septum may be heralded by recurrence of chest pain, rapidly developing right heart failure, intense dyspnea and increasing shock.[71]

2. Pathologic Physiology

a. Perforation of the intraventricular septum is nearly always a consequence of occlusions of both the anterior and posterior descending arteries. The usual sequence is for one occlusion to be old and one to be recent.[13] This deprives most of the septal myocardium of its normal blood supply.
b. As the AV node and bundle of His are usually deprived of normal blood supply by this type infarction, it is not surprising that complete heart block is so often seen in patients who eventually have septal rupture. Bundle branch block and nodal rhythm[71] are often associated with ruptured septum, before or after rupture.

RUPTURE OF PAPILLARY MUSCLE

1. Incidence and Prognosis

a. Both papillary muscles of the left ventricle attach to the leaflets of the mitral valve. The mitral valve requires papillary muscle support to function properly. Papillary muscle rupture therefore creates a severe hemodynamic abnormality, with relative mitral insufficiency, manifesting as rapidly developing dyspnea and pulmonary edema.[13]

b. In a few selected instances of relative mitral insufficiency due to papillary muscle weakness, operations have been successful, with mitral valve replacement.

Thromboembolism

The 2 types of thromboembolic phenomenon which may occur with acute myocardial infarction are systemic embolism and pulmonary embolism.

SYSTEMIC EMBOLISM

There is a tendency for blood to clot on the injured surface of the left ventricle. These clots may remain in the chamber as mural thrombi, or they may leave the heart and go as emboli to the systemic arterial circulation. If they leave the heart, they may go to the brain, the abdomen or the extremities, where they will probably cause necrosis distal to the site in the arterial vascular tree where they lodge. The probability of mural thrombi dislodging and becoming systemic emboli is greater if there is an arrhythmia. Treatment of systemic emboli in acute coronary care is limited by the preexisting acute condition of the patient and must therefore be individualized. One or more of the following therapeutic steps may be carried out, depending on the clinical condition of the patient before and after peripheral embolization.

1. Anticoagulation.
2. Conversion of arrhythmia.
3. Sympathetic nerve block—if the embolus is in an extremity.
4. Vasodilators.
5. Surgical removal of embolus under some circumstances.

PULMONARY EMBOLISM

Those emboli arising from the deep veins of the legs, which dislodge and find their way to the lung to cause pulmonary infarction are the commonest of thromboembolic phenomena. Emboli are responsible for 8% of the deaths in acute myocardial infarction.[125] Massive pulmonary embolism has been found to be 1 of the 3 most common causes of sudden death in acute myocardial infarction, the other 2 being arrhythmias (the most com-

mon) and rupture of the heart. Pulmonary emboli may well go unrecognized in the situation of acute myocardial infarction. However, with a change in the site and character of chest pain, cough and particularly bloody sputum, pulmonary embolus must be considered. The lactic dehydrogenase level may rise, but it may also rise in acute myocardial infarction.

Symptoms of Pulmonary Infarction:

1. Dyspnea.
2. Pleurisy.
3. Cough or hemoptysis.
5. Tachypnea.
5. Tachycardia.
6. Fever.
7. Pleural friction rub.
8. Splinting of thorax.
9. Elevated lactic acid dehydrogenase level.
10. Infiltrate on x-ray.
11. Location by radioisotope lung scan.
12. Acute cor pulmonale, made manifest by clinical symptoms, including shock, and ECG changes.

Therapy

1. Oxygen.
2. IV heparin sodium.
   a. IV heparin is part of the immediate therapy for major pulmonary embolism. In addition to its anticoagulant action, heparin may help reverse bronchospasm after acute embolization.
   b. It is probable that the antibronchospasm effect is initially more important than the anticoagulant effect.
   c. Doses of 7,500–10,000 units are administered every 4 hours. This dosage is higher than that usually recommended for anticoagulation, and there is evidence that the higher initial dosage reduces mortality.
3. Isoproterenol (Isuprel)[176] is recommended for the hypotension that frequently occurs with pulmonary embolism. Dosage is 4 mg. isoproterenol diluted in 1 L. of 5% D/W.
4. If blood pressure does not respond to isoproterenol, the use of vasopressor agents such as norepinephrine (levarterenol; Levophed) is advised.
5. Pulmonary embolectomy is a last desperate measure. Persistent shock is the chief indication for the surgical procedure of pulmonary embolectomy. Results, even in patients without acute myocardial infarction, have been disappointing.

CHAPTER 7

Complications Not Immediately Life Threatening

Pericarditis

INCIDENCE

In 30–80% of autopsied patients with acute myocardial infarction, pericarditis has been noted.[71,118] The bedside diagnosis of pericarditis is much less common, being made in perhaps 20% or less.

DIAGNOSIS

1. Pain may be difficult to diagnose, since it may be confused with the pain of almost any condition, such as:
   a. An extension of acute myocardial infarction or the prolonged pain of acute myocardial infarction.
   b. Pneumonia.
   c. Intra-abdominal conditions.
2. Pain may be pleuritic in character (increased by deep inspiration) or constant. If the pain is constant, it may be severe and unrelenting for the first 24–36 hours, requiring frequent doses of narcotic analgesics for relief. The pain usually changes intensity with changes in position. It may be slightly relieved by sitting upright and leaning forward. If pericarditis is on the diaphragmatic surface, the pain may be referred to the supraclavicular area.
3. Friction rub is present in 20% of the cases of pericarditis. The rub lasts from a few hours to 2 weeks but may be very transient.
4. Electrocardiographic changes frequently occur with pericarditis but may be confusing in the presence of changes caused by the acute infarction. Comparison of electrocardiograms with the recent abnormal records showing the acute infarction may be valuable.
5. Pericarditis occurs between the first and tenth day following acute myocardial infarction, 80% occurring on days 2 to 4.

THERAPY

1. Analgesics for pain.
2. Reassurance.
3. Steroids have been advocated. However, most clinicians feel steroids are not usually necessary.
4. The question occurs as to whether to discontinue anticoagulants.
   a. Usually anticoagulants are not discontinued.
   b. Discontinuation of anticoagulants should be done or considered if there is:
      1) Widespread friction rub.
      2) Ventricular aneurysm.
      3) Pericardial effusion.
5. If cardiac tamponade occurs, pericardiocentesis may be lifesaving.

PROGNOSIS

Localized pericarditis in acute myocardial infarction has little or no bearing on recovery as a general rule.

Pneumonia

Pneumonitis is a relatively frequent complication of acute myocardial infarction. The pathologic physiology of acute myocardial infarction includes decreased cardiac output, pulmonary vascular engorgement (congestion) and frequently some degree of transudate into the alveoli of the lungs, providing an excellent medium for bacterial growth. With stasis due to inactivity and decreased ventilation due to narcotics administered for pain, there are excellent predisposing conditions for the growth of bacteria normally present in the pharynx.

Some degree of pulmonary vascular engorgement frequently occurs in the presence of the decreased cardiac output of acute myocardial infarction; and it is impossible to detect the occurrence of even moderate amounts of pulmonary vascular engorgement by stethoscopic examination. Therefore, it is impossible to predict in which patients with "uncomplicated" acute myocardial infarction pneumonitis will develop. It is necessary that careful clinical observation be carried out by the physician and nurse on each patient with acute myocardial infarction.

The use of prophylactic antibiotics is debated. Prophylactic antibiotic therapy is used by some with the rationalization that the fever, tachycardia and toxicity caused by the pneumonitis are of greater risk to the patient than is a toxic reaction to an antibiotic or the emergence of bacterial resistance. Careful clinical observation would seem preferable to prophylactic antibiotic therapy.

If pneumonitis is detected, attempts should be made to determine the causative organism by sputum smears and cultures. Therapy should be instituted with one of the broad-spectrum antibiotics while awaiting the results of bacteriologic examination.

The choice of antibiotic agents and the route of therapy will depend upon the clinical circumstances at the time the pneumonitis is detected.

Gastric Dilatation and Paralytic Ileus

Gastric dilatation and/or paralytic ileus are most often manifested by abdominal distention and/or vomiting. They are most likely to be seen in diaphragmatic infarction, particularly in the presence of diaphragmatic pericarditis. However, other factors are definitely involved and diaphragmatic infarction is not the only situation in which acute gastric dilatation and/or paralytic ileus may occur in a patient with acute myocardial infarction.

Gastric dilatation and paralytic ileus are detected by careful clinical observation and, if necessary, x-ray examination. Both complications are treated by inserting a nasogastric tube into the stomach and applying continuous suction. Acute gastric dilatation may predispose to rapid clinical deterioration, and it should be kept in mind as a possible precipitating factor when other causes are not immediately apparent. The probability of gastric dilatation occurring is increased in the presence of complications of acute myocardial infarction, particularly cardiogenic shock, thus adding to the severity of the complication.

Electrolyte loss via the nasogastric tube must be evaluated and appropriate replacement made at frequent intervals in order to avoid fluid–electrolyte imbalance.

Urinary Retention

Urinary retention is most apt to occur in elderly males who have pre-existing prostatic hypertrophy and partial mechanical bladder neck obstruction. The obstruction becomes complete after admission to the acute coronary care unit where enforced bedrest and administration of narcotics and other drugs take place. Urinary retention may, of course, occur in female patients and in younger patients of both sexes. It is treated by inserting an indwelling catheter. The usual precautions for catheter insertion and care should be carried out. An indwelling catheter may also be necessary in the event of immediate life-threatening complications of acute myocardial infarction, most particularly cardiogenic shock, in which frequent measurement of urinary output may be necessary. The question of prophylactic antibiotic therapy after insertion of an indwelling catheter has been debated.

Postmyocardial Infarction Syndrome

Postmyocardial infarction syndrome[1,14,118] occurs in about 3% of the patients with acute myocardial infarction. This complication is due to pleuropericarditis and usually occurs 2–12 weeks after infarction.

Symptoms of fever, pericarditis, pleuritic pain, pericardial or pleural effusion (frequently hemorrhagic), pericardial friction rub, arthralgia, elevated sedimentation rate, increased white blood cell count, and occasionally ECG changes of pericarditis are observed.

It seems that this syndrome represents a tissue reaction to cardiac damage in susceptible individuals.

The syndrome is usually self-limiting, lasting 1–4 weeks, and is usually treated with aspirin, or if necessary with steroids. The course is sometimes lengthy with remissions in symptoms and relapses. The pain must be distinguished from that due to an extension of myocardial infarction and the patient reassured.

As the effusions in this syndrome may be hemorrhagic and thus may cause cardiac tamponade, anticoagulant therapy following onset of the syndrome should be discontinued unless strong indications are present for their use.

PART II

Therapeutic Measures, Procedures and Pharmacologic Agents for Acute Coronary Care

CHAPTER 8

General Therapeutic Measures

Introduction

It has been estimated that in the future coronary care units will save over 100,000 lives annually. This figure represents about 20% of the half million Americans who currently die each year from acute myocardial infarction. It is significant that, if it occurs, this dramatic change will not be achieved by more efficient resuscitation of patients with cardiac arrest. It will be accomplished by *preventing* these cardiac arrests, whether they be due to arrhythmia or the other "immediate life-threatening complications" of acute myocardial infarction.

This chapter deals with the general medical care and atmosphere for the patient in the coronary care unit. It deals in particular with the general care of the patient as this care relates to the prevention of major complications of acute myocardial infarction. The general therapeutic measures covered are those not specifically discussed as such elsewhere. There are a number of seemingly minor aspects of acute coronary care which must be taken into consideration. These apparently minor aspects considered cumulatively have significant bearing on the comfort, the occurrence of complications and the ultimate well-being of the patient with acute myocardial infarction.

It may be that adequate consideration and attention to these numerous seemingly minor details will prevent the onset of one of the serious life-threatening complications of acute myocardial infarction. It is not possible, of course, to prevent all complications of acute myocardial infarction. Among the most common fatal complications of acute myocardial infarction in the past have been the cardiac arrhythmias. Some of the general therapeutic measures stressed to help in *prevention* of cardiac arrhythmias are the following.

1. Control of pain, anxiety and distress.
2. Control of congestive heart failure, pulmonary edema, shock, hypoxia and acidosis.

3. Avoidance of the following:
   a. Iced drinks.
   b. The Valsalva maneuver (use laxative, no bedpans; no straining at stool, use bedside commode).
   c. Rectal interference (avoid taking temperature rectally, rectal examinations).
   d. Pulmonary embolism (wrap legs; turn frequently; exercise legs; correct congestive heart failure).

The foregoing conditions to be avoided and/or controlled involve essentially all of the "immediate life-threatening complications" of acute myocardial infarction.

The entire purpose of hospital treatment is to prevent the complications of acute myocardial infarction while helping the patient through a safe hospital stay and convalescence. This chapter is therefore concerned with the less tangible aspects of acute coronary care which cumulatively add to a more positive control of the patient's environment and bodily functions, both physical and mental.

Control of Pain

Narcotic Analgesics for Pain

The one symptom which most frequently draws the attention of patient and physician alike to the possibility of acute myocardial infarction is pain. A review of patients hospitalized for acute myocardial infarction in a community hospital over a 4-year period[216] revealed that essentially all patients suspected of acute myocardial infarction at the time of hospital admission received narcotic analgesics for pain and anxiety.

Patients having pain severe enough to bring them to medical attention usually require narcotic-analgesic medications initially for pain relief. The pain associated with acute myocardial infarction usually results in severe anxiety and should be treated promptly with adequate doses of effective drugs. The drugs most commonly used at present are: morphine, meperidine (Demerol) and pentazocine (Talwin). Specific information regarding these drugs and their effects will be found under Narcotics and Analgesics in Chapter 14.

Morphine may be given in doses of 10–15 mg. every 2–4 hours, and occasionally more often if severe pain warrants. Atropine may be necessary to block the vagal effects of morphine and should readily be administered if vagal effects occur. Atropine is administered concomitantly with morphine by some clinicians. Meperidine in doses of 75–125 mg. may be effective, but it may cause significant parasympatholytic effects, with resultant tachycardia. Pentazocine has been used with encouraging results[95,96] and has the advantage of being a so-called non-narcotic drug.

OXYGEN FOR PAIN AND THERAPY

1. Oxygen is usually administered routinely during the first 24–48 hours to the patient with uncomplicated acute myocardial infarction.[266]
2. Oxygen should be administered routinely as long as significant pain persists.
3. Oxygen therapy should be reinstated if pain recurs. (Recurrent pain may indicate progressive myocardial damage and therefore may be a bad prognostic sign, however, the pain of acute pericarditis may be confused with the recurrence of pain associated with myocardial damage.)
4. Oxygen therapy should be reinstituted or continued in the presence of pulmonary infarction, shock, heart failure, pulmonary edema, cyanosis, dyspnea or Cheyne-Stokes respiration.
5. Caution must be exercised in patients with chronic lung disease and pulmonary insufficiency.

PROLONGED PAIN

1. Pain that continues after 48 hours may be due to another infarction, extension of previous infarct, pulmonary embolus or pericarditis.
2. The prognosis in the presence of intractable pain is not good, as one of the above complications may be the cause.
   a. Intractable pain may require repeated administration of narcotic analgesics.
3. Coronary pain may be confused with angina early in the course of acute myocardial infarction. As angina represents temporary ischemia and coronary pain represents prolonged ischemia, the 2 cannot occur in the same patient early in the course of acute myocardial infarction by definition. However, the character of pain may be similar in a patient with pre-existing angina.
   a. Nitroglycerin will relieve the pain of angina but is contraindicated in the first week after acute myocardial infarction. It is also contraindicated in the presence of hypotension, since nitroglycerin may itself cause hypotension or the precipitation of hypotension.

Control of Anxiety

INTRODUCTION

There is excellent reason to believe that psychic stress, particularly in the presence of acute myocardial infarction, may be important in the pathogenesis of arrhythmias and circulatory failure.[108] Therefore, it is desirable to keep psychic stress to a minimum. This is accomplished by soothing the anxious patient and attempting to avoid situations stressful to the patient.

PATHOLOGIC PHYSIOLOGY

Emotional disturbances have been found to have a profound effect on the circulation, causing changes in heart rate, cardiac output, blood pressure, tone of peripheral vessels and the ECG. These cardiovascular changes have been found particularly likely to occur in the emotional state which may develop in persons who find themselves in a *hazardous situation*.[59] This stress has an effect on circulation similar to that caused by small doses of epinephrine. It is apparent that even the most uninitiated patient would feel himself in a hazardous situation when placed in the coronary care unit, with electronic equipment about him and personnel in greater numbers per patient than might ordinarily be anticipated in the hospital at large.

The nurse and other coronary care unit personnel are in the most advantageous position to help calm the apprehensive patient.

ANXIETY FROM PAIN

Anxiety is also caused by the pain associated with acute myocardial infarction and is controlled with narcotic-analgesics and/or sedative agents.

ANXIETY AFTER PAIN

Control of anxiety after the pain disappears is usually accomplished by using a sedative, hypnotic or tranquilizer. The drug most familiar to the individual physician is probably the drug of choice in this situation. Librium (chlordiazepoxide), Valium (diazepam), Thorazine (chlorpromazine) and Sparine (promazine) have been suggested.[15] However, because of their alpha sympathetic blockade effects, chlorpromazine, promazine and related phenothiazines should be used with caution in the patient with acute myocardial injury. The drug of choice is undoubtedly quite individual to the patient.

NURSING ROLE

1. **Attitude.** The general attitude of the nurse toward

the patient in the coronary care unit and what she is to tell that patient are well covered in numerous other sources (see references in the Introduction of this manual). In general, the nurse should be cheerful, reassuring and truthful without enumerating possible fatalities or complications.

2. **What to tell the patient.** Each physician has his own thoughts as to what and how much the patient should know, and his decision is undoubtedly tempered by the psychic stability of the patient and numerous other factors. The nurse must ascertain the attitude of the attending physician with regard to these matters.

3. **Visitors.** The visiting hours are, of course, restricted in the coronary care unit for numerous reasons. If it is noted that a patient gets acutely upset, either visibly or as manifested by increased pulse rate, when a specific individual is present or during discussion of a specific subject, this fact should be brought to the attention of the attending physician and steps taken to remedy the situation.

Diet and Fluids

DIET

For the first few days after acute myocardial infarction the diet should be liquid or soft, low in calories and easily digestible. It has been theorized in the past that large amounts of rich foods increased the circulation to the stomach and therefore indirectly removed circulatory capacity available to the heart. This assumption was based on the fact that many acute myocardial infarctions occurred immediately after large and rich meals or during the digestive period for such a meal. Whether this be the situation or not, low calorie, liquid or soft feedings are undoubtedly preferable because they would be less likely to precipitate the complication of gastric dilatation or paralytic ileus than would a "regular" diet.

Hot or *cold* liquids should not be allowed the patient during the first days (and perhaps weeks) following acute myocardial infarction, as they cause vagal stimulation and therefore increase the possibility of cardiac arrhythmias.

FLUIDS

In all patients admitted to the acute coronary care unit with suspected acute myocardial infarction it is advisable to cannulate a vein so that intravenous medication may be given immediately should an emergency situation arise, and so that fluids may be administered as needed. In some instances this will be via a continuous intravenous drip through a plastic cannula; in other instances the venous route will be obtained using a plastic cannula with an obturator so that IV fluids need not be attached.

Among the numerous therapeutic applications of fluids in acute myocardial infarction are the use of dilute solutions for intravenous infusion in various complications of acute myocardial infarction; maintenance of daily insensible loss, and replacement therapy for losses via other routes. The uses and indications for fluid and electrolyte therapy are beyond the scope of this manual.

Many clinicians feel central venous pressure (CVP) monitoring should be carried out on all patients with acute myocardial infarction. This is accomplished via a "long-line" IV catheter.

Rest and Extent of Exercise

FORMER TREATMENT OF ACUTE MYOCARDIAL INFARCTION

For a number of years acute myocardial infarction was treated with absolute bed rest for several weeks. This procedure was based primarily on the fact that autopsy findings showed that a time period of 6–8 weeks was required for complete scarring of an acutely infarcted area of myocardium. More recently there is a trend toward more liberal use of some degree of ambulation. As mentioned further under Bowel and Bladder Control and Care, the bedside commode is frequently utilized when patients have no complications and in poor-risk patients who are not in shock.

MODIFIED "ARMCHAIR" TREATMENT

Activity may be carried slightly further, permitting several daily periods of sitting up in a chair; this is often referred to as "armchair" treatment.[60] Some modification of this regimen is used by many physicians, when feasible. It is felt that modified "armchair" treatment and modified ambulation to bedside commode or private bathroom provides the following advantages:
1. An increase in mental and physical comfort.
2. Easier pulmonary ventilation, therefore a decreased risk of hypostatic pneumonia.
3. A decrease in risk of peripheral venous stasis with thrombosis and embolism.
4. A lower incidence of urinary retention and severe constipation.

It was originally thought that the patient should be lifted and transported from bed to chair with an absolute minimum of effort on his part.[60] It would seem that a reasonable objective in any form of modified "armchair" treatment would be that the *increase* in work load imposed upon the heart should be at a minimum. This can frequently be accomplished by lowering the bed to a level at which the patient may place his feet directly on the floor and by aiding him to his feet. Careful instructions should be given the patient, emphasizing that he move to the bedside commode, chair or private bathroom at a slow gait.

PREVENTING THROMBOEMBOLISM

Whether modified "armchair" treatment is used or not, an attempt should be made to gain the advantages of that type treatment. A patient remaining at bed rest, and in particular the poor-risk, elderly, obese patient with venous insufficiency or peripheral edema, should have the legs wrapped with elastic bandages or be equipped with adequate elastic stockings. All patients should be encouraged to move the toes and feet actively to prevent venous congestion and also to turn from side to side and to breathe deeply at frequent intervals. Absolute bed rest results in a "deconditioning" of the patient, with decreased muscle tonus and loss of postural compensatory stability (causing postural hypotension).

MODIFYING THE PROGRAM

The general personality of the patient as well as the severity of the illness, complications and numerous other factors will affect achievement of the general goals mentioned previously.

Numerous programs for rest and extent of exercise are possible in patients with acute myocardial infarction. The best results and the best program for each patient are likely to occur if the physician and nurse keep the general objectives in mind, evaluate the patient individually and proceed on a highly individual basis. Attempts to institute rigid, routine orders should be avoided.

Anticoagulation

Anticoagulant therapy is usually carried out in the presence of acute myocardial infarction. Frequently anticoagulant therapy is started with heparin, and therapy with one of the coumarin derivatives is often begun at the same time. As sufficient anticoagulant action occurs from the coumarin derivative, heparin is gradually decreased. Anticoagulant therapy is routinely given by many physicians in the absence of contraindications to that therapy. The question of long-term therapy in acute myocardial infarction is still under debate. However, short-term therapy during the acute phase is generally accepted, in the absence of contraindications. (See Anticoagulation Therapy, Chapter 11.)

Anticoagulant therapy is given to prevent thromboembolism, particularly in poor-risk patients. There has been no evidence to date that it otherwise beneficially alters the course of acute myocardial infarction.

Anticoagulation once started is nearly always continued until 6–8 weeks postinfarction.

Bowel and Bladder Control and Care

THE VALSALVA MANEUVER[97]

The Valsalva maneuver is a physiologic maneuver familiar to all of us though we may not be aware of its name or of its significance in acute myocardial infarction. The Valsalva maneuver is performed whenever any type of "straining" is accomplished. It is important in acute coronary care, in that it occurs with straining at stool, straining to micturate and the straining to lift oneself off the bed or to climb off and on the bed, particularly when using the familiar bedside footstool.

Mechanism of Valsalva Maneuver

The Valsalva maneuver is performed by:
1. Voluntary closure of the glottis.
2. A strong expiratory effort.
3. Contraction of the abdominal muscles.
4. Accompanied by marked increase in intrathoracic and intra-abdominal pressures.

Circulatory Changes

Circulatory changes brought about by the Valsalva maneuver during expiratory effort:
1. Return of blood from the head and extremities is impeded by increased intrathoracic and intra-abdominal pressure.
2. Venous pressure in the head and extremities rises abruptly.
3. Venous blood is withheld from the thoracic cavity by the change in pressure gradient, thus temporarily decreasing the blood return to the heart.
4. As a result, cardiac output decreases and pulse pressure decreases.
5. With decreased aortic pressure as a result of decreased cardiac output, pressor-receptors in the carotid sinus and aortic arch are activated and cause a reflex increase in heart rate.

Circulatory changes with relaxation of expiratory effort are the following.
1. The impeded venous blood surges into the heart.
2. As a result of increased venous return the heart forcibly ejects the blood into the greater and lesser circulations.
3. The systemic output abruptly increases, causing an increase in the blood pressure.
4. The increased blood pressure activates the aortic and carotid sinus pressor-receptors, bringing about a period of reflex bradycardia.

Over-all Changes of Valsalva Maneuver

It can be seen that the Valsalva maneuver can alter the hemodynamics of the patient in several important ways. The pulse rate is increased, the blood pressure is transiently increased, then the pulse rate is decreased. These hemodynamic changes are, of course, much more apt to cause complicating difficulties in an already injured cardiovascular system than in a well patient.

When the ECG monitor is observed while a patient

goes through the Valsalva maneuver, these changes can frequently be observed in vivid fashion.

Causes of Valsalva Maneuver

1. Straining at stool due to constipation.
2. Straining to urinate.
3. Straining to raise up in bed or to get in or out of bed, particularly in getting up and down bedside steps.
4. Grunting due to pain.

BOWEL CARE AND CONTROL

Bowel care is important. Constipation is liable to occur in the patient with acute myocardial infarction due to enforced rest, altered diet, medications administered for pain and other causes. It is important to prevent constipation since constipation leads to excessive utilization of the Valsalva maneuver in the process of straining at stool.

1. The Bedside Commode

Most authorities currently recommend the use of a bedside commode or of a bathroom, if readily available, for bowel movements and frequently for urination at certain stages of acute coronary care. The sitting position helps prevent the strain of the Valsalva maneuver, which is associated with the use of the cold bedpan, and the associated anxiety and distress caused by the abnormal positioning for its use as well as the embarrassment many patients experience from using the bedpan.

Many coronary care units currently being built are equipped with remote monitoring attachments in private bathrooms provided for each patient.

2. Methods for Preventing Constipation

　　a. Cathartics (see Chapter 16). Many physicians prescribe gentle laxatives from the first day in the coronary care unit.
　　b. Avoidance of bedpans by use of bedside commode or private bathroom facility.
　　c. Advising the patient particularly not to strain at stool in order to prevent excesses of the Valsalva maneuver.

BLADDER CARE AND CONTROL

Various aspects of bladder control and care may present difficulties in management. The following are some of the abnormalities which may occur.
1. The necessity for catheterization of the patient with acute cardiogenic shock.
2. Pre-existing bladder neck contracture and/or prostatic hypertrophy with mechanical obstruction of the outlet and straining, with concomitant Valsalva maneuver in ordinary voiding.

3. Urinary retention due to medications. Atropine in the high doses required for certain bradycardias nearly always causes urinary retention, requiring catheterization.

If insertion of a catheter is required, it is probably preferable to insert an indwelling catheter. Catheterization is also necessary when accurate intake and output determinations must be carried out, particularly in the incontinent patient. The question of antibiotic prophylaxis during catheterization is still under debate. However, many physicians utilize prophylactic antibiotics in the already ill patient to retard the possibility of genitourinary tract infection with secondary gram-negative septicemia.

Other Therapeutic Measures

POTASSIUM, GLUCOSE AND INSULIN

Effects of Hypopotassemia (Hypokalemia, Low Potassium)

It has been definitely proved that patients with potassium deficiency have a much higher incidence of ectopic beats and AV conduction disturbances than patients who have normal serum potassium levels.[43,224-227] This is true whether the serum potassium deficiency is associated with causes unrelated to the cardiovascular system, is related to diuretic response or is related to toxicity from digitalis with or without diuretics.

Potassium, Glucose and Insulin in Treatment of Myocardial Infarction

Much investigation has been carried out on glucose, insulin and potassium in prophylactic therapy of acute myocardial infarction, with the accumulation of a considerable amount of evidence in favor of its use.[79,145,150,251] Methods of intravenous therapy, oral therapy and combinations of the 2 have been used. Contraindications have been set forth.

An IV method utilizes 1,000 ml. of 10% D/W, 40 mEq. potassium and 20 units of regular insulin.[150] A method of oral therapy has also been used.[79,145] There are those who doubt the proved effectiveness of this "polarizing" therapy and feel it is potentially harmful.[61]

Polarizing Therapy in Prevention of AV Block

It is felt by some that polarizing therapy helps in prevention of AV block in acute myocardial infarction.[79,145] It is also felt that the rate of infusion of IV polarizing solutions may have considerable bearing on the over-all statistical results.

It is difficult adequately to evaluate the use of polarizing solutions and methods of therapy at present because of the large number of variables to consider.

Hyperbaric Oxygenation in Treatment

The use of oxygen under higher than normal atmospheric pressures would seem to have a reasonable place in the treatment of acute myocardial infarction. To date not enough study has been carried out to have statistically valid results for this type of therapy.[80]

CHAPTER 9

Antiarrhythmic Therapeutic Agents

Many drugs have antiarrhythmic activity. This consideration of antiarrhythmic agents will deal with those drugs most commonly used in acute coronary care, their electrophysiologic actions, indications and pharmacophysiology. These agents exert their antiarrhythmic effects either directly on tissues or through the autonomic nervous system (see Chapters 14 and 15).

It must be remembered that almost any arrhythmia may be observed in abnormalities of the central nervous system and have indeed been produced experimentally by stimulation of various portions of the central nervous system (see also Central Nervous System Control in Chapter 2). Therefore, the beneficial action of sedation, particularly in the presence of acute myocardial infarction, should not be ignored.

The following is a consideration of the individual agents and procedures utilized in treating arrhythmias.

Atropine

DESCRIPTION

Atropine is a parasympatholytic agent which inhibits the actions of acetylcholine (ACh) on structures innervated by the postganglionic cholinergic nerves and inhibits the effects on smooth muscles that respond to the acetylcholine but lack cholinergic innervation.

ACTIONS (PHARMACOPHYSIOLOGY)

1. The exact mechanism of atropine blockage of cholinergic response is unknown, but it is *not* through prevention of the release of acetylcholine. The net effective mechanism of action of atropine is via blockage of the parasympathetic receptors, with subsequent prevention of uptake of the acetylcholine which is released from the parasympathetic nerve endings. The increased functional refractive period of the AV node produced by excess vagal stimulation is blocked by atropine: thus the drug has an effect on heart block as well as on sinus bradycardia.
2. The main effect of atropine on the heart is to alter the rate. With average clinical doses of 0.4–0.6 mg., the rate may be *temporarily* decreased, probably due to stimulation of the medullary vagal nuclei. The slowing is rarely marked, and there are no accompanying changes in blood pressure or cardiac output. There is also some dryness of mouth, inhibition of sweating and mild dilatation of the pupils. This decreased rate is usually followed by an *increase* in heart rate. The desired effect of atropine as used in the coronary care unit is to block the effects of the vagus nerve and is, therefore, opposite to that of vagal stimulation. (See Autonomic Nervous System in Chapter 2.)
3. With larger doses (1 mg.) there is a progressively increasing tachycardia caused by blocking vagal effects on the SA pacemaker. This effect is sometimes preceded by slowing.
4. Use of atropine in clinical treatment of bradycardia associated with acute myocardial infarction has resulted in an increased heart rate and arterial blood pressure, along with obvious general clinical improvement in some patients.
   a. The amount of elevation of heart rate reflects the degree of vagal tone under which the patient was functioning prior to atropine injection.[231]

METABOLISM

Atropine disappears rapidly from the blood and is distributed throughout the entire body. Much is destroyed by enzymatic hydrolysis, particularly in the liver, and some is excreted by the kidney unchanged.

INDICATIONS

In acute coronary care atropine is utilized in the treatment of bradyarrhythmias. (See Bradyarrhythmias in Chapter 4.)

CONTRAINDICATIONS

Glaucoma, asthma and benign prostatic hypertrophy are contraindications. For necessary use of atropine in

67

acute coronary care, these are relative contraindications.

DOSAGE AND ADMINISTRATION

See Bradyarrhythmias in Chapter 4.

TOXICITY

Toxic effects are related to the parasympatholytic effect of the drug and include speech disturbance, difficulty in swallowing, restlessness and fatigue, headache, dry skin, hot skin, difficulty in micturation, rapid pulse, iris practically obliterated, blurred vision, ataxia, hallucinations, delirium and coma. The severity is dependent on the dose that has been administered.

Diphenylhydantoin (Dilantin)*

DESCRIPTION

Diphenylhydantoin (DPH) was introduced some 30 years ago for the control of epileptic seizures. It was not until 1965 that its use for therapy of arrhythmias prompted enough study to begin evaluating its cardiovascular effects. Diphenylhydantoin is analogous in structure to the barbiturates.

MECHANISM OF ACTION (PHARMACOPHYSIOLOGY)

1. Primary action of DPH is a stabilizing action against repetitive stimuli. This results in an "antispreading effect" from any area of abnormal discharge.
   a. The stabilizing action of DPH has been shown to be common to all excitable membranes.
2. The actions of DPH appear to be due to its direct action on the myocardium and the conduction system and not to effects on reflexes from the central nervous system.
3. The antiarrhythmic effect of DPH may result from its ability to alter transmembrane ion flux.
   a. The total exact electrophysiologic mechanism has not been elucidated. However, some excellent work has been done on canine Purkinje fibers, with some results that do not fit our previous thoughts on the mechanism of action of antiarrhythmics.[232]
   b. It is safe to conclude that the consistent effects of DPH on the myocardium and conduction system of the heart are not yet completely known.
4. DPH directly *depresses* myocardial function via the following:
   a. Reduction in myocardial contractility (negative inotropism).
   b. Rapid IV administration of DPH has resulted in a more marked negative inotropic effect than slow injection.

---

*References: 7, 10, 18, 77, 100, 184, 231–235, 241, 245.

c. Repeated IV injections have produced cumulative negative inotropic effects.
5. DPH exerts specific vasodilating effects when given IV, with decreased central aortic pressure.
6. It may increase coronary blood flow and decrease coronary resistance.
7. It has many effects similar to those of quinidine and procainamide.
8. DPH decreases ventricular automaticity.
9. It depresses the sinus node.
10. AV block in man and animals is increased.[233,234]
11. In correctly administered clinical doses, DPH does not cause significant changes in cardiac output, peripheral resistance or pulmonary vascular pressures.

METABOLISM[100,231]

1. Diphenylhydantoin is detoxified by the liver and excreted as the glucuronide via the bile into the intestinal tract. A small amount is excreted directly in the feces. A greater part is reabsorbed from the intestinal tract into the blood stream and excreted in the urine.
2. After a single IV dose there is an hourly decline of 10% in the plasma level.
3. The metabolites are excreted in the urine within 48 hours.
4. At all dosages, tissue concentrations are generally higher than plasma levels.

INDICATIONS

1. Diphenylhydantoin is used principally in ventricular arrhythmias and more particularly for digitalis-induced arrhythmias.
2. Indications for use of DPH are precisely the same as those for propranolol (p. 77 f.), except that DPH has no effect on atrial fibrillation and atrial flutter.

CONTRAINDICATIONS

1. Hypotension and shock.
2. Heart block and bradycardia.
3. Overt heart failure.
4. Severe myocardial disease.

PRECAUTIONS

1. Inject SLOWLY.
2. Monitor electrocardiograph and blood pressure.
   a. There is a tendency toward shortening of the PR interval; no change is seen in the QRS complex; there is a shortening of the QT interval.[235]
3. Possibly its effect is enhanced by phenobarbital.
4. There is variable effect on AV conduction.
5. DPH will not convert atrial fibrillation or flutter.

DOSAGE AND ADMINISTRATION

1. Diphenylhydantoin may be administered by the oral, IM or IV route.
2. It is available as 100 mg. capsules and as a powder which can be dissolved for IV or IM use.
3. IV administration. The dose is not finally determined to date, but:
   a. It should not exceed 5–10 mg./kg. in a single dose.
   b. It should be administered in dilute solution in not less than 5 minutes, and preferably over 10–15 minutes.
   c. Convenient dose of 250 mg. given over 5 or more minutes is an effective, predictable and safe dose. (Maximum speed of administration should be 1 mg./kg./minute.)
   d. Effective in 4–10 minutes.
   e. Larger doses (10–15 mg./kg.) have been given IV, but only over several hours.
   f. Blood concentration associated with a beneficial effect is approximately 10–20 μg./ml.[231]
   g. DPH solution is alkaline and may cause pain at the injection site.
4. Oral administration.
   a. DPH is absorbed almost quantitatively from the gastrointestinal tract.[100]
   b. Dosage 200–400 mg./day.
   c. Peak effect may take several days to occur via oral administration.

TOXICITY AND SIDE EFFECTS

Cardiovascular Toxicity

1. Toxicity is related to cardiovascular action of the drug.
   a. Depression of left ventricular function.
   b. Vasodilatation.
   c. Depression of sinus node.
2. Bradycardia and high degrees of heart block with resultant hypotension are seen.
3. In critically ill patients rapid administration has resulted in respiratory and cardiac arrest.
4. Studies show cardiovascular-depressing effects of DPH depend not only on dosage but also on rapidity of administration, when given IV.
   a. Small doses given rapidly cause undesirable results.
   b. Larger dose may be tolerated when given over a longer period.

Noncardiovascular Effects

1. Central nervous system changes—drowsiness, depression, nervousness, ataxia, nystagmus, tremor, visual disturbances.
2. Also transient nausea, light headedness, headache.
3. Gingival hypertrophy.
4. Arthralgia.

5. Skin—pruritus, morbilliform and urticarial eruptions.
6. Eosinophilia, pancytopenia, megaloblastic anemia, syndrome resembling infectious mononucleosis.

Drug Interactions

1. DPH decreases the inotropic effect of digitalis preparations and sympathomimetic amines. This effect is via its general myocardial depressant effects.[245]
2. DPH interferes with the effects of corticosteroids (e.g., dexamethasone) almost immediately after administration, probably via the chemical structure of DPH.[241]

Therapy of Toxicity

1. Discontinue DPH when significant signs or symptoms of toxicity occur.
2. Hypotension: discontinue DPH; administer vasopressors if hypotension is not rapidly corrected by discontinuing the drug.
3. Sinus bradycardia or AV block may be rapidly reversed with atropine 0.4–1 mg. IV.

Isoproterenol (Isuprel)[†]

GENERAL

Isoproterenol is a synthetic catecholamine, sympathomimetic amine, beta adrenergic stimulating drug (beta sympathomimetic) structurally related to norepinephrine and epinephrine.

PHYSIOLOGIC ACTIONS

The physiologic actions of isoproterenol are almost exclusively beta sympathomimetic. The drug has almost no action on alpha receptors.

Cardiovascular Effects

1. Inotropic effects. Isoproterenol has a significant inotropic action.[131]
   a. Increases cardiac output.[7,10,72,86]
   b. Increases ventricular systolic force.[72,160]
   c. Increases stroke output.[72,86]
   d. Decreases left ventricular end-diastolic volume and pressure.[86]
   e. Decreases left ventricular mean volume.[86]
      1) Via more effective emptying.
   f. Increases left ventricular ejection rate.[160]
   g. Decrease in the afterload to contraction.[86]
   h. Increase in myocardial uptake of oxygen out of proportion to pressure–time (tension) index.[86]
      1) Probably via increased rate of fiber shortening.
   i. Augments both ventricular excitability and automaticity, making the infarcted heart more susceptible to arrhythmia.[75]

[†]References: 7, 10, 72, 75, 86, 131, 160, 176.

j. Even with greater myocardial work, no evidence of anaerobic myocardial metabolism is found with IV infusion in man.
2. Chronotropic effect.
   a. An increase in cardiac rate.[7,10,72]
3. Coronary artery effects.
   a. An increased coronary artery blood flow.[86]
   b. A decreased coronary artery resistance.[7,86]
      1) Via marked coronary vasodilatation.
   c. An increase in oxygen content of coronary venous blood.[86]
4. Vascular resistance.
   a. Isoproterenol markedly decreases systemic vascular resistance.[7,10,72,160]
      1) IV infusion lowers peripheral vascular resistance, mainly in the skeletal muscle and cutaneous vascular beds, but also in the renal and mesenteric vascular beds.
      2) Usual doses in man generally increase cardiac output enough to overcome the decreased peripheral vascular resistance and to maintain or raise systolic pressure.
      3) Larger doses (1 μg./kg.) in man cause a striking fall in blood pressure.
   b. The usual therapeutic doses in man do not change pulmonary blood pressure.

Other Effects

1. Isoproterenol constricts veins by acting on beta receptors in dogs and possibly in man.[7] This action increases venous return to the heart.
2. It relaxes smooth muscle of the bronchial tree, thus acting as a bronchodilator.
3. It increases total body metabolism[160] as determined by oxygen consumption.

METABOLISM

Isoproterenol is considered to be metabolized and eliminated by the same routes as epinephrine and to have approximately the same duration of action.

INDICATIONS

1. Used in bradyarrhythmias (see Bradyarrhythmias in Chapter 4).
   a. Sinus node dysfunction, via stimulation of sinus pacemaker.[10]
   b. Second-degree AV block. Improves AV conduction.[10]
   c. Complete AV block. Increases ventricular excitability and automaticity.[72,75]
2. Treatment of cardiogenic shock (see Chapter 5).
   a. Used for its beta sympathomimetic effect (see Physiologic Actions).
3. Treatment of pulmonary emboli[176] (see Thromboembolism in Chapter 6).
   a. Bronchodilator effects.

b. Cardiac effects in this situation.
   c. Given by IV infusion.
   d. Used in conjunction with IV heparin.
4. Bronchodilation in bronchial asthma or bronchospastic conditions, when not contraindicated.

CONTRAINDICATIONS

1. Do not use in patients with tachycardia caused by digitalis toxicity.[10]
2. Avoid use with other sympathomimetic amines *simultaneously* as these agents all cause cardiac stimulation. Additive effect would result.
   a. May be used in carefully controlled clinical conditions with careful monitoring of electrocardiograph.
   b. May be administered by *alternating* with other sympathomimetic amines.
3. Administer with caution in patients:
   a. With diabetes mellitus.
   b. Sensitive to sympathomimetic amines.
   c. With hyperthyroidism.
4. Administer carefully in the face of hypovolemia, as severe hypotension may result due to the decrease in peripheral vascular resistance.
   a. Volume expanders (dextran of low molecular weight) may be administered in conjuntion with isoproterenol.
      1) The dextran infusion significantly increases the stroke volume and cardiac output in experimental cardiogenic shock treated with isoproterenol.[75]

ADMINISTRATION AND DOSAGE

Isoproterenol is readily absorbed when given parenterally or as aerosol. Absorption is unreliable when given sublingually or orally.

Clinically, the most effective and controlled method of administration is by IV infusion.

IV Administration

1. In bradyarrhythmias.
   a. Dosage is 2 mg. isoproterenol in 500 ml. of 5% D/W. Solution contains 4 μg./ml.
   b. 5 ml. ampule contains 1 mg. isoproterenol.
   c. Administer 1.0–1.5 ml./minute (4–6 μg./minute) until desired effects are obtained or toxic effects are seen.
   d. Infuse at above rate until heart rate is increased to approximately 60/minute, then titrate to maintain.
   e. If ventricular irritability occurs, use lidocaine simultaneously. Use bolus followed by infusion.
   f. See also Bradyarrhythmias in Chapter 4.
2. In cardiogenic shock.
   a. IV dosage is 1 mg. per 500 ml. of 5% D/W. Solution contains 2 μg./ml.

1) Titrate to raise blood pressure—may need to use volume expander.
2) In shock, heart rates above 130 beats/minute attributed to isoproterenol predispose to ventricular arrhythmia.

3. Precautions.
   a. Monitor with electrocardiograph to regulate dosage.
   b. Observe for ectopic ventricular activity; if it occurs, treat with lidocaine.

TOXIC EFFECTS

1. Serious reactions, other than ectopic ventricular activity, are frequently seen.
2. The following reactions have been reported.
   a. Flushing of the face.
   b. Sweating.
   c. Mild tremors.
   d. Nervousness.
   e. Headache.
   f. Tachycardia with palpitations, manifested as a sensation of pounding in the chest.
   g. Weakness.
   h. Nausea.
3. Reactions disappear quickly with decrease of infusion rate and usually do not require discontinuation of isoproterenol treatment.
4. Cumulative effects are not reported.
5. In a *few* patients paradoxically precipitated Adams-Stokes seizures during normal sinus rhythm or transient heart block have been reported.

Lidocaine (Xylocaine)‡

DESCRIPTION

Lidocaine is a rapid-acting local anesthetic agent which has not yet been approved for cardiovascular use by the federal Food and Drug Administration. The drug has had wide utilization in the treatment of cardiac arrhythmias in coronary care units.

Lidocaine is available commercially as the soluble hydrochloride salt of the base lidocaine in 1 and 2% solutions under the trade name Xylocaine.

When used in the coronary care unit lidocaine is always administered intravenously.

ACTIONS (PHARMACOPHYSIOLOGY)

Mechanism of Action

Local anesthetic agents generally prevent the generation and conduction of nerve impulses. The drugs act on the cell membrane, where they affect the permeability to sodium and potassium ions.

Lidocaine given IV has rapid action via rapid diffusion

‡References: 3, 7, 15, 17, 19, 44, 45, 47-53, 55-58, 75, 103, 104, 170, 171, 239.

to and penetration of cell membranes. It is rapidly metabolized by the liver. Thus, careful control can be maintained over duration of action of the drug via IV administration.

Cardiovascular Effects

Significant cardiovascular pharmacophysiologic effects of lidocaine administration are:
1. Decreased myocardial irritability.
2. Increase in the stimulation threshold of the ventricle during diastole.[47]
3. Prolonged conduction time.
4. Prolonged depolarization time.
5. No significant change in the duration of the *absolute* refractory period.[47]
6. Prolonged *effective* refractory period.
7. Very little depression of the SA node.
8. Potent peripheral vasodilating action in larger doses (causing hypotension).[17]
9. No significant decrease in cardiac output in patients not suffering acute myocardial infarction.[239]

Hemodynamic Effects and Dosage

With the IV administration of a bolus of lidocaine, all parameters of cardiac and vasotonic function are initially slightly depressed. These functions return to normal levels within 3–5 minutes.[51] In appropriate doses these effects are minimal, and it is generally agreed that the vasodilating action (and thus the hypotensive effect) of lidocaine is less than that of procainamide (Pronestyl). However, blood pressure should be closely monitored while lidocaine is being administered.

It has been found in man that the blood pressure, heart rate and QRS durations are not adversely affected by single or adequately spaced multiple doses of 1–2 mg./kg. of lidocaine.[55,239] No lasting hemodynamic effects can be observed clinically in man at lidocaine doses of 1–1.5 mg./kg.[49,58] and these doses are *usually* adequate to suppress the arrhythmias treated with this drug. In a few normal dogs lidocaine at 2.0 mg./minute caused no changes in stroke volume, heart rate, left ventricular systolic pressure or left ventricular end-diastolic pressure.[75] It has been found that no significant clinically lasting hemodynamic effects are noted with a 50 mg. bolus of lidocaine for the average 70-kg. patient, and minimal effects occur with a 100 mg. bolus of lidocaine. However, at higher dosages some depression of ventricular function does occur transiently and usually without symptoms.[53] In a few patients, low or high doses of lidocaine have been followed by a transient decrease in arterial blood pressure.[53]

METABOLISM

Lidocaine is rapidly removed from the blood stream by the liver, where it is metabolized by amidases to form free and conjugated phenols. These metabolites as well as approximately 10% of the unchanged lidocaine are excreted by the kidney.[103,104] Lidocaine action dissipates within 10–20 minutes.

CHOICE AS THERAPEUTIC AGENT

Lidocaine has been found to be an excellent antiarrhythmic agent for ventricular ectopic arrhythmias for the following reasons.
1. It can be administered in large enough doses to suppress ventricular arrhythmias with minimal side effects.
2. It has rapid onset of action.
3. It can be administered as a bolus or by constant IV infusion.
   a. The fastest way to achieve sustained therapeutic effect is to deliver a bolus IV and follow immediately with a constant IV infusion.[3,44,48,171]
   b. If the bolus is effective, constant infusion has been found necessary to maintain the antiarrhythmic effect.
4. It has a short half-life of approximately 20 minutes in the blood stream[55] (i.e., it is rapidly cleared from the blood stream).
5. Toxic side effects disappear rapidly when the administration of lidocaine is discontinued.

INDICATIONS

Lidocaine has demonstrated antiarrhythmic effects in the following situations:
1. Ventricular premature contractions.
2. Ventricular tachycardia.
3. Digitalis-induced ventricular arrhythmias.[49]
   a. Used as premedication in cardioversion of digitalis-induced ventricular tachycardia.[19]
4. Supraventricular ectopic beats (auricular premature contractions, nodal premature contractions) but *not* supraventricular tachycardia or auricular fibrillation. [44,45,49]
5. Ventricular irritability following electric shock conversion (defibrillation) of ventricular fibrillation.
6. As a regular premedication for (or immediately following) emergency cardioversion.
   a. Used as a bolus followed by IV infusion.
   b. Used as routine premedication for elective cardioversion.

CONTRAINDICATIONS AND PRECAUTIONS

Contraindications to administration of lidocaine are associated with heart block, liver disease and hypotension. They include:
1. Atrial tachycardia with heart block.
2. Hypotension and heart block.
3. Heart block with bradycardia.
   a. Slow nodal or idioventricular pacemaker.

   b. Unless pacemaker electrode catheter has been inserted into the right ventricle.
4. Give with caution in the presence of *liver disease* since lidocaine is 90% metabolized by the liver.
5. Precaution: All patients receiving IV lidocaine should be monitored for blood pressure and ECG change.

DOSAGE AND ADMINISTRATION

Instituting Rapid Therapy[3,44,45,48,50,52,56,171]

1. Initially administer IV bolus of 1–2 mg./kg.
   a. Ventricular irritability usually decreases within 45–90 seconds.
2. Follow bolus with IV infusion of lidocaine of 1–2 mg./minute.
   a. 2,000 mg. (2 Gm.) of lidocaine are mixed to total 500 ml. of 5% D/W, giving a concentration of 4 mg./ml. This is then administered via microdrip technique to control the rate of infusion.[15]
   b. Other dosage strengths (in mg./ml.) may be prepared and substituted, if a low fluid volume per given time interval is desired.
3. The IV drip of lidocaine should be given no longer than 4–5 days.
   a. If necessary, change to IM or oral procainamide before decreasing and terminating lidocaine infusion.

Repeated Bolus Technique

1. Lidocaine boluses of 0.5–2 mg./kg. have been given at 3–20 minute intervals.[15,46.54]
   a. Do not exceed a maximum of 4 such doses, since toxic symptoms are usually manifest above this dosage.
   b. IV infusion should be started if multiple boluses are necessary.

Limits of Dosage

1. Titration should be carried out to the point required to prevent ventricular irritability.
2. It has been found that patients do not generally respond to continuous lidocaine infusions of less than 1 mg./minute.[48]
3. Toxic symptoms may occur at infusion rates over 4 mg./minute; they appear to be avoidable if dosage is kept below 4 mg./minute for the average 70-kg. patient.[48]
   a. Serious toxic symptoms usually occur when the dosage rate is 5 mg. or more per minute for the average 70-kg. patient.
   b. Stupor and seizures have been found to occur at high dosage infusion rates of 8 mg./minute.[48]
4. The total amount of lidocaine administered in a single hour should not exceed 400–500 mg.[2]

5. If the patient is not responding to lidocaine therapy in adequate dosage look for the presence of one or more of the following conditions:
    a. Acidosis.
    b. Hypoxia.
    c. Electrolyte abnormality.
    d. Occult heart failure.
    e. Hypotension.

Blood Levels

1. Lidocaine blood levels 5 minutes after injection of a single dose of 1 mg./kg. varied from 0.3 to 1.8 μg./ml. The variations were inversely proportional to body weight in man[55] (i.e., high weight, low blood level and vice versa). This suggests that the dose of lidocaine should be weight related.
2. Initial antiarrhythmic effect in man occurred with blood levels of 0.6–1.2 μg./ml.

TOXIC AND SIDE EFFECTS

Most Severe Toxic Effects

The sites of toxic and side effects may be seen in the cardiovascular or the central nervous system. The major, most severe side effects are:[48]
1. Central nervous system depression.
2. Convulsions.
3. Hypotension.

Central nervous system depression occurs to some degree with all dosages of lidocaine. Most patients receiving the lidocaine bolus followed by IV infusion in appropriate clinical doses to suppress ventricular arrhythmias manifest some degree of lightheadedness. As the dose of lidocaine is increased with relationship to the patient's individual tolerance, additional central nervous system symptoms arise, such as euphoria and confusion, and if the dose becomes high enough convulsions may occur. Lidocaine also has indirect stimulating effects on the central nervous system.[103]

Large doses of lidocaine cause peripheral vasodilation and myocardial depression with hypotension. With very high doses, hypotension and respiratory arrest may occur due to medullary (brain stem) depression.

Toxic effects are related to (1) the dosage administered in a given time interval and (2) the size of the patient. The effects of lidocaine given IV have been determined experimentally and clinically in man.

Specific Toxic Symptoms from IV Therapy

1. Toxic effects at low blood levels include:
    a. Euphoria.[57,103]
    b. Lightheadedness.[49,103]
    c. Confusion.[57,103]
    d. Blurred or double vision.[103]
    e. Headache.[49]
    f. Sweating.[103]
    g. Discomfort in breathing, speaking or swallowing.[49,103]
    h. Sensations of heat, cold or numbness.[103]
    i. Heaviness in the chest different from cardiac pain.[103,170]
    j. Slurred speech.[49]
    k. Tinnitus.[49]
    l. Muscular fasciculations or twitching.[103]
2. Toxic effects at higher levels in the blood are:
    a. Extreme apprehension.[103]
    b. Disorientation.[103]
    c. Convulsions, generally preceded by definite EEG changes.[103]
        1) Petit mal.[57]
        2) Grand mal.[57]
        3) Focal seizures.[56]
3. Toxic effects at extremely high blood levels are:
    a. Cardiovascular depression[103] with decreased cardiac output.[44]
    b. Hypotension[56,58] via the following:
        1) Central nervous system medullary depression.
        2) Myocardial depression.
        3) Peripheral vasodilatation.
    c. Respiratory arrest[103] via central nervous system medullary depression.
    d. Bradycardia.[44]

Discussion

1. Drowsiness is the only significant side effect found at carefully controlled clinical doses of 1.5 mg./kg. initial bolus followed by 1–2 mg./minute infusions administered to man in clinical settings.
2. A great deal of experimental work has been done on laboratory animals to correlate blood levels with measurable toxic side effects.
3. Extremely large doses have been found to produce a marked fall in blood pressure,[44,48] bradycardia and decreased cardiac output in experimental animals.
4. Experiments in laboratory animals using various IV doses comparable to those used clinically for cardiac arrhythmias produced no measurable side effects.[51] In the same study, doses 8 times greater than the dose level utilized clinically in man to suppress ventricular arrhythmias were given, and there was found to be a measurable, but transient and relatively small, detrimental effect on cardiovascular function, which returned to normal in a short period.
5. It has been found that convulsions have definitely occurred in man at levels above 5 mg./minute for the average 70-kg. patient. Usually those measured rates at which convulsions occur have been from 6.5 to 8 mg./minute infusion rates. It should be noted that this extremely high level is essentially never *intentionally* used clinically in man.
6. The ECG is a poor guide to the toxic effects of lidocaine, but in extremely high doses early ECG signs are impaired AV conduction (heart block) and intra-

ventricular conduction (widened QRS complex). This widened QRS complex may be significant of toxicity when it exceeds 25% of the original QRS width.[15]

Therapy

1. Central nervous system depression. At the first sign of toxicity dosage should be decreased; if more severe effects occur, the infusion must be stopped.
2. Convulsions. These are treated with IV barbiturates (Pentothal sodium or amobarbital sodium) or diazepam (Valium).
3. Hypotension. Treat with vasopressors. Since this hypotension is most probably via depressed cardiac output, central and peripheral sympathetic nerve blockade and central nervous system medullary depression, a combined alpha and beta stimulating sympathomimetic such as Levophed might be desirable.

COMMENT

There is basic agreement that lidocaine is in many ways superior to procainamide for IV therapy of ventricular arrhythmias, in that (1) hypotension occurs less often with IV lidocaine than with IV procainamide and (2) lidocaine is more effective in controlling arrhythmias in clinical settings. The more effective clinical control of arrhythmias is probably due to the tendency to use more effective doses of lidocaine than procainamide since the occurrence of hypotension is less probable during IV administration of lidocaine.

As lidocaine is administered only by the IV method, it is usually desirable to start procainamide IM or orally in doses of 500–1,000 mg. every 4–6 hours. It may be desirable to start this therapy immediately upon starting the lidocaine or it may be more desirable to have the arrhythmia under treatment with one agent at a time. This is a matter of clinical judgment at the time. When procainamide therapy is begun, the lidocaine dose is decreased by increments, maintaining suppression of ectopic activity.

Procainamide (Pronestyl)§

DESCRIPTION

Procainamide is a derivative of the local anesthetic agent procaine and is qualitatively similar to procaine in both chemical structure and pharmacologic actions. Procainamide differs from procaine chemically only in the replacement of the ester linkage of the procaine molecule by the amide structure of procainamide. The advantage of the amide over the parent procaine compound depends upon:

1. The more favorable ratio between the cardiac and central nervous system activities of procainamide.

§References: 7, 10, 26, 46, 47, 67, 101, 102, 125, 236.

a. Procainamide has less central nervous system effect.
2. The amide not being as readily hydrolyzed by plasma esterases and therefore having a longer duration of action.

ACTIONS (PHARMACOPHYSIOLOGY)

Mechanism of Action

The mechanism of action of procainamide is qualitatively similar to that of lidocaine. There is general agreement that the mode of antiarrhythmic action of procainamide is probably related to the drug's effect on the cardiac cell membranes and the flow of ions across the membrane during depolarization and repolarization. This is essentially the same mechanism of action as that of lidocaine.

Cardiovascular Effects

Significant cardiovascular pharmacophysiologic effects of procainamide administration are as follows:
1. Decreased myocardial irritability.
   a. Diminished excitability to faradic electric current.[46,101]
2. Decreased force of myocardial contraction.
3. Decrease in vasomotor tone.
   a. The combination of decreased myocardial contraction and vasomotor tone may cause hypotension.
   b. A single IV infusion of procainamide will produce a significant decrease in cardiac output and arterial pressure in patients with cardiac disease but will cause almost no change in patients with normal hearts.
   c. Procainamide-induced hypotension is more common in patients with an already lowered blood pressure due to primary heart disease; the hypotension appears to be dose related.
      1) This indicates the need for care in the use of procainamide in the presence of acute myocardial infarction, and particularly in the presence of impending or actual cardiogenic shock.
4. Increase in the stimulation threshold of the ventricle during diastole.[47]
5. Prolonged conduction time throughout the heart.
   a. Procainamide slows conduction in the atrium, atrioventricular junctional tissue and ventricle. This is noted in the ECG as prolongation of the PR interval and QRS duration. This is a normal function of procainamide.
   b. The ECG effects are not necessarily regarded as manifestations of toxicity, but rather as manifestations of the effects on cardiac muscle essential to the action of the drug.
      1) When the increase in QRS is over 25% of the initial time interval, it becomes significant and is considered to indicate toxicity.

6. Decreased frequency of pacemaker impulse activity.
7. No significant change in duration of the *absolute* refractory period.[47]
8. Prolonged *effective* refractory period.
   a. The refractory period of the atrium is considerably more prolonged than that of the ventricle.[101]

METABOLISM

Procainamide is less readily hydrolyzed than procaine, and plasma levels decline slowly. The decrease in plasma levels is approximately 10–20% an hour. Other sources suggest the half-life is 3–4 hours.[258] The drug is excreted primarily in the urine. About 10% is excreted as free and conjugated para-aminobenzoic acid and about 60% as the unchanged form. The fate of the remainder is unknown.[101]

At plasma levels of 10–20 mg./L. (levels within a range of therapeutic concentration for patients *without* acute myocardial infarction), only about 15% of the drug is bound to plasma proteins, but considerable amounts are reversibly bound to various organ tissues. This explains in part the *relatively* slow decline in plasma levels, since tissue depots of the drug serve as a reservoir as the drug is lost by excretion or metabolic transformation.[101]

Other sources describe the level suppressing active ventricular arrhythmias in acute myocardial infarction as 4–6 mg./L.[258]

INDICATIONS

1. Supraventricular ectopic beats.
   a. Atrial premature contractions.
   b. Nodal premature contractions.
2. Control of auricular arrhythmias, particularly if recently developed.
   a. Atrial fibrillation of short duration may be converted to normal sinus rhythm.
3. Ventricular premature contractions (VPCs).
4. Digitalis-induced ventricular extrasystoles (not therapy of choice).
5. Ventricular tachycardia (not therapy of choice).

CONTRAINDICATIONS AND PRECAUTIONS

Absolute Contraindications

1. Patients with complete AV heart block.
2. Hypersensitivity to the drug. Cross-sensitivity to procaine and related drugs must be borne in mind.
3. In patients with myasthenia gravis.

Precautions

1. In patients receiving normal dosage who have both liver and kidney disease, drug accumulation may produce symptoms of overdose.
   a. Principal overdose symptoms are ventricular tachycardia and severe hypotension.

2. Patients with renal damage alone or with congestive heart failure excrete procainamide more slowly than do normal persons and accumulative effects are more probable.
3. Monitoring of ECG and blood pressure is necessary when IV procainamide is administered, due to the possible development of AV block, ventricular tachycardia or hypotension.
   a. If the ECG shows evidence of impending heart block, discontinue IV administration at once.
   b. If the ventricular rate is significantly slowed by procainamide, without attainment of regular AV conduction, administration should be stopped and the patient re-evaluated. (AV block may have developed.)
      1) Asystole may result from continued procainamide administration under this circumstance.
   c. If, when administering the drug in atrial fibrillation or flutter, the ventricular rate should suddenly increase as the atrial rate is slowed, the drug should be discontinued. (AV block may have developed or increased.)
4. Caution is required in the following situations.
   a. Marked disturbances of AV conduction, such as partial AV block or bundle branch block.
   b. Severe digitalis intoxication.
   c. Procainamide in the above situations (a and b) may result in additional depression of conduction with the occurrence of ventricular asystole or fibrillation.
5. Contraindications and precautions for procainamide should be exercised in all situations in which they would apply to lidocaine, as the effect of the 2 drugs is approximately the same, except for a greater likelihood of hypotension and arrhythmias with procainamide.

ADMINISTRATION AND DOSAGE

Choice of Therapeutic Agent

1. Procainamide is an excellent antiarrhythmic agent for ventricular ectopic arrhythmias. However, by the IV route, procainamide in adequate therapeutic dosage appears to be somewhat more toxic than lidocaine due to its tendency to cause hypotension.
2. The effects of procainamide are more beneficial in ventricular than in atrial arrhythmias.
3. Procainamide has an advantage over lidocaine in that it may be administered orally, IM or IV. However, if the drug is to be utilized in *acute situations*, IV infusion is usually the most acceptable form. The other routes have great advantage in maintenance therapy.

Routes of Administration

1. Intravenous infusion.
   a. *Limited to extreme emergency situations*, such as arrhythmias in acute coronary care.

b. Widening of the QRS complex and widening of the PR interval are normal effects of procainamide on the conduction mechanism. The occurrence of these increases, therefore, does not necessarily mean toxicity has occurred. However, a QRS increase of more than 25% of the pretreatment value has been found to correlate with clinical cardiovascular toxicity. If this situation occurs, infusion should be temporarily discontinued.

2. Intramuscular administration.
   a. Hypotension seldom occurs when this route of administration is used.[102]
   b. After IM administration, plasma levels occur fairly rapidly. After absorption, plasma levels of the drug decline at a rate of 10–20%/hour. The half-life is 3–4 hours when hepatic and renal functions are normal.[258]

3. Oral Administration.
   a. Hypotension rarely occurs with oral therapy.
   b. The drug does not accumulate on repeated oral dosage. Thus, dosage schedules of 500–750 mg. every 4–6 hours may be used. (See also Procainamide Prophylaxis in Chapter 4.)
   c. Absorption of procainamide from the gastrointestinal tract is rapid and virtually complete; the peak plasma level of the drug is achieved usually within less than 2 hours after oral administration.[7,10]

Dosage

1. IV infusion (seldom used in acute coronary care).
   a. Administered at a rate not exceeding 25–50 mg./minute, with a dose range of 0.2–1 Gm. being required per 6-hour period.
   b. Dilute solutions must be used.
   c. IV infusion should be monitored by the ECG so that the infusion may be stopped if:
      1) Arrhythmia is interrupted.
      2) An excessive widening of the QRS complex or prolongation of the PR interval with an increase over 25% of original values occurs, as this increase has been found to correlate well with clinical cardiovascular toxicity.
   d. The patient should be kept in a supine position and blood pressure measurements made almost continuously.
      1) If blood pressure falls more than 15 mm. Hg, infusion should be temporarily discontinued.[7,10]

2. IM administration.
   a. Dosage of 0.5–1 Gm. repeated at 4–6 hour intervals until oral therapy is feasible.
   b. It has been determined that the dose must be at least 750 mg. every 6 hours to achieve an effective blood level.[125] A dosage range has been recently proposed for prophylaxis based on body weight.[258] It would seem that this might apply also to active therapy.

3. Oral administration.
   a. Doses of 0.5–1 Gm. at 4–6 hour intervals may be given.
   b. Suggested dosage for ventricular extrasystoles is 0.5–0.75 Gm. every 4–6 hours.
   c. For atrial arrhythmias, initial dose is 1.25 Gm., followed in 1 hour by 0.75 Gm. If there are no ECG changes, a dose of 0.5–1 Gm. may be given every 2 hours until arrhythmia is interrupted or limits of toxicity reached. (Procainamide is not the primary therapy of choice.)
   d. Suggested maintenance dose is 0.5–1 Gm. every 4–6 hours.
   e. IM and oral doses are the same since absorption is virtually complete by either route.

Toxic Effects

1. In considering the toxic and side effects of procainamide, as well as contraindications and precautions, the chief source of informational reference for anticipating these factors is the pharmacophysiologic action of the drug. The accentuation or acceleration of certain cardiovascular conditions can be predicted and anticipated by keeping in mind these actions of the drug.
2. See also Contraindications and Precautions. Most important immediate toxic effects are AV block, ventricular tachycardia and hypotension.
3. Hypotension due to procainamide via IV administration is frequently observed in unanesthetized subjects and regularly observed in anesthetized subjects. It has been thought to be due mostly to peripheral vasodilatation, but observations on myocardial contractility indicate that decreased contractility may contribute significantly to the hypotension.[101]
4. Patients receiving digitalis and procainamide have had episodes of second-degree AV block.[26] These usually subside when both drugs are temporarily discontinued.
5. With IV administration, serious disturbance of cardiac rhythm, such as ventricular asystole and fibrillation, have occurred.
6. One investigator[26] reported fever as the commonest side reaction in the therapy of VPCs with procainamide. Chills may also occur.
7. When the drug is given orally the most frequently observed untoward effects are anorexia, nausea and vomiting. These symptoms may also occur with parenteral administration.
8. Other symptoms include flushing, a bitter taste, diarrhea, weakness, mental depression, giddiness and psychosis with hallucinations.
9. Drug rashes, lymphadenopathy and eosinophilia have occurred.
10. Agranulocytosis has been reported with *long-term* administration of high doses.

11. A syndrome resembling systemic lupus has been increasingly reported with *long-term* administration[7,67,236] (L. E. prep positive).

COMMENT

It appears obvious that, when used *intravenously,* procainamide in clinically effective dose levels is somewhat more toxic than lidocaine for the same uses. This toxicity is particularly manifest as hypotension. It would seem, therefore, that Xylocaine given by IV infusion initially for the immediate treatment of certain arrhythmias is the drug of choice. This may then be followed by intramuscular or oral procainamide. Procainamide may also be added to Xylocaine therapy for the treatment of resistant arrhythmias, when necessary.

Oral and IM procainamide causes fairly rapid blood levels and the drug is completely absorbed by both routes. Therefore, supplementing of lidocaine therapy, instituting maintenance therapy or changing from lidocaine to procainamide therapy may be readily done without IV use of the drug.

New dosage schedules for oral administration based on body weight and more frequent administration have recently appeared[258] and additional definitive work will undoubtedly be done in the near future.

Propranolol (Inderal)||

DESCRIPTION

Propranolol is a beta adrenergic blocking agent (betasympatholytic) and is similar in chemical structure to isoproterenol (the most potent beta adrenergic stimulating agent).

ACTIONS

Mechanism of Action

1. Propranolol has antiarrhythmic effects attributable to 2 separate mechanisms of drug action. These are:
   a. Beta adrenergic blockade effects.
   b. Direct myocardial effects similar to those of quinidine and procainamide. These effects are independent of the beta-blocking action and occur at different dose levels.
2. Propranolol exerts its beta adrenergic blocking action by competitive inhibition. The propranolol molecule occupies the receptor sites that would normally be occupied by the adrenergic agent, thus competing for that beta adrenergic site and preventing the adrenergic agent from occupying the site. This inhibits the action of the adrenergic agent at the receptor sites.
   a. The chemical structural similarity to isoproterenol undoubtedly relates to the ability of the propran-

olol molecule to fit into the beta receptor site.
3. The beta receptor blockade occurring by competitive inhibition explains the following drug interactions; since these drugs do not mediate their action by adrenergic stimulation, their effects are not blocked by propranolol.
   a. Cardiac effects of digitalis, calcium and the xanthines are not abolished by propranolol.
   b. Vasodilating effects of nitroglycerin and acetylcholine are not blocked by propranolol.
   c. Propranolol blocks catecholamine-induced release of free fatty acids and glycogenolysis.

Cardiovascular Effects

1. For antiarrhythmic effects, see Mechanism of Action above.
2. Heart rate is decreased.
3. Cardiac output is decreased.
4. All indexes of left ventricular function are decreased; thus:
5. Myocardial oxygen consumption is significantly reduced.
6. Systemic arterial pressure may be reduced.
7. Pulmonary arterial pressure and total pulmonary vascular resistance are elevated.

METABOLISM

Pharmacologic and metabolic half-life of IV propranolol is in the range of 40–60 minutes. There is wide tissue distribution in animals.

INDICATIONS

The potency of propranolol in reducing cardiac function makes it imperative that it be used in clinical situations in which myocardial function is not greatly compromised by the disease. Indications for use must be carefully weighed against the cardiovascular depressant properties of the drug.

There is little sympathetic nervous system activity in normal subjects resting in the supine position, and beta adrenergic blockage produces little effect. In the presence of acute myocardial infarction the situation is quite different[68] and a small dose of propranolol has been shown to produce dramatic responses. A dose of 5 mg. IV in patients with acute myocardial infarction has been seen to cause decreased heart rate, increased circulation time, decreased systolic arterial pressure and decreased cardiac output (via decreased rate without significant changes in stroke volume[185]—i.e., without compensatory increase in stroke volume usually seen when the heart rate decreases). This is potentially quite hazardous.

Propranolol has been used to treat arrhythmias and digitalis-induced arrhythmias. The chief area of use in acute myocardial infarction is in digitalis-induced arrhythmias.

||References: 7, 15, 18, 68–70, 92, 184–186, 189, 230, 269.

Arrhythmias, not Necessarily in Acute Myocardial Infarction

1. Atrial fibrillation and flutter—slows ventricular response.
2. Paroxysmal atrial tachycardia—good prophylaxis.
3. Nodal tachycardia.
4. Premature atrial contractions.
5. Ventricular tachycardia, when cardioversion techniques are not available.
6. Ventricular premature contractions.
7. Slowing of sinus tachycardia. (*Note*: Sinus tachycardia is not an arrhythmia.)

Digitalis-Induced Arrhythmias

1. Supraventricular tachycardia with block.
2. Nodal tachycardia.
3. Premature atrial contractions.
4. Ventricular tachycardia, in conjunction with cardioversion.
5. Ventricular premature contractions.
6. Ventricular fibrillation (prophylaxis).

CONTRAINDICATIONS AND PRECAUTIONS

1. Overt heart failure.
2. Compensated heart failure, not digitalized.
   a. Propranolol may be used in appropriate instances when the patient is on therapeutic doses of digitalis. (*Note*: Cardiac inotropic digitalis effect is *not* blocked by propranolol.)
3. History of heart failure.
4. Severe myocardial disease.
5. Heart block and bradycardia.
6. Hypotension of cardiogenic shock.
7. Severe pulmonary hypertension.
8. Acute and chronic obstructive pulmonary disease.
   a. Bronchial asthma and emphysema.
9. In patients prone to hypoglycemia, including labile diabetics.
10. Use with caution in presence of impaired renal or hepatic function.
11. In patients on adrenergic-augmenting psychotropic drugs (including MAO inhibitors) and during the 2-week withdrawal period for such drugs.
12. In patients receiving catecholamine-depleting drugs, such as reserpine and methyldopa.

DOSAGE AND ADMINISTRATION

1. Oral administration.
   a. Dose 10–30 mg. 3 times daily, preferably given on an empty stomach.
   b. Maximum effects in 1–4 hours.
   c. Effects present for 5–6 hours.
   d. Titrate dosage.
2. IV administration.

a. Dose 1–3 mg. IV, rate of administration not to exceed 1 mg./minute.
b. Slow administration is mandatory due to myocardial-depressing effects.
c. Monitor ECG and blood pressure during administration.
d. Discontinue drug when desired alteration in rate or rhythm is noted.
e. Discontinue if toxic effects appear.
f. If there is no response to initial dose, a second dose may be carefully administered after 3 minutes.
g. If the second dose yields no response, no additional medication should be given for 4 hours.
h. Total IV dose of 10 mg. at one time should not be exceeded.

TOXIC EFFECTS

Cardiovascular Toxicity

1. Sudden death has occurred after IV administration.
2. Hypotension may follow either oral or IV use.
3. Bradycardia, partial heart block and complete heart block have occurred.
4. Increased total pulmonary vascular resistance may accentuate right heart failure.
5. Frequently congestive heart failure has worsened or has been precipitated.

Extracardiovascular Toxicity

1. Incidence is infrequent, with less than 2% of patients receiving the drug manifesting symptoms of toxicity.
2. Peculiar feeling of lightheadedness.
3. Visual disturbances.
4. Gastrointestinal symptoms.
5. Purpura, nonthrombocytopenic or thrombocytopenic (very rare).
6. Patients with obstructive pulmonary disease may have further decreased pulmonary function via increased airway resistance.
7. Implicated as cause of hypoglycemia in diabetic patients.

Therapy of Toxic Side Effects

1. Stop administration if there are indications of decreased cardiac function.
2. Stop drug if other toxic effects occur.
3. If congestive heart failure occurs, *administer* therapeutic doses of *digitalis*. (*Note*: Digitalis is not blocked by drug.)
4. Hypotension is treated by discontinuing drug and administering vasopressors (to overcome beta adrenergic blockade).
5. Bradycardia is treated with IV atropine, 0.3–1 mg.

COMMENT

Although propranolol may be beneficial in selected patients, the routine administration of a beta-blocking agent to all patients with acute myocardial infarction is contraindicated, since it does not prevent arrhythmias or recurrence of pain and has no influence on mortality.[186-189] The drug may precipitate the serious clinical states of cardiac failure, pulmonary edema, hypotension and bradycardia, with associated development of the shock syndrome.[68]

Quinidine

DESCRIPTION

Quinidine[7,10,125,169] is the dextrorotary isomer of quinine and one of the natural alkaloids found in cinchona bark.

ACTIONS (PHARMACOPHYSIOLOGY)

Mechanism of Action

The mechanism of action of quinidine is essentially the same as that of procainamide and lidocaine of the local anesthetic group of drugs. Quinidine and procainamide are qualitatively similar in their cardiovascular actions, though quantitatively different. The systemic toxic effects of quinidine and procainamide are quite different.

Cardiovascular Effects

The cardiovascular effects of quinidine are the same as those of procainamide except for quantitative differences, as mentioned above.

Quinidine is generally regarded as a *strong myocardial depressant*. Quinidine depresses excitability, conduction velocity and contraction of the myocardium.

In addition to its direct effects upon the heart, there is some indirect effect resulting from an anticholinergic action. The anticholinergic activity of quinidine prevents slowing of the heart rate produced by direct reflex vagostimulation or by cholinergic drugs. Clinically, sinus tachycardia may result from the anticholinergic action of quinidine.

METABOLISM

After being absorbed, quinidine is rapidly bound to the plasma albumin. When total plasma concentration of the drug is within the therapeutic range (3–6 mg./L.), approximately 6% of the quinidine is in the bound form. Substantially all of the drug administered is excreted by the kidney, with about 10–15% appearing in the urine within 24 hours as unchanged quinidine.

INDICATIONS

Choice of Agent

Quinidine is never the agent of choice in the presence of acute myocardial infarction. Except in very difficult situations or when quinidine must be added as a supplement to already instituted therapy to convert or control an arrhythmia, quinidine is seldom, if ever, a drug of choice in the emergency antiarrhythmic therapy situations arising with acute myocardial infarction.

Specific Indications

Because of the relative toxicity of quinidine, this drug has not been and probably will not be extensively used in acute coronary care. Therefore, little can be said of its use in such care. Quinidine has had utilization in both atrial (auricular) and ventricular arrhythmias in cardiac patients with various types of heart disease and arrhythmias but *NOT* suffering acute myocardial infarction.

In the patient without acute myocardial infarction, quinidine has been used in the following situations:
1. Atrial fibrillation.
2. Atrial flutter.
3. Paroxysmal supraventricular tachycardia.
4. Premature systoles.
5. Ventricular tachycardia.

CONTRAINDICATIONS AND PRECAUTIONS

Most contraindications to quinidine are relative. Each patient's needs should be considered individually.
1. An absolute contraindication is that of complete AV block with either AV nodal or idioventricular pacemaker, as these pacemakers may be suppressed by quinidine.
2. Extreme caution must be exercised in administration of quinidine to patients with incomplete AV block, as complete block and asystole may be produced.
3. Special caution must be exercised in the presence of digitalis intoxication.
   a. Overdose of digitalis may result in bradyarrhythmias.
   b. Quinidine is specifically contraindicated in digitalis intoxication manifest by AV conduction disorders.
4. An absolute contraindication is a history of thrombocytopenia purpura associated with previous quinidine administration.

DOSAGE AND ADMINISTRATION

Routes of Administration

Quinidine administration may be oral, IM or IV.
1. Oral administration.

a. Quinidine is essentially completely absorbed after oral administration.

b. Maximal effect occurs within 1–3 hours and persists for 6–8 hours.

c. When cumulative effects are sought, repeated dosage is given at intervals of 2–4 hours.

2. IM administration.
Quinidine is given intramuscularly as quinidine gluconate and yields peak effects in 30–90 minutes.

3. IV administration.
Intravenous administration does not produce instantaneous effect; accordingly, the drug should be administered slowly and cautiously when given IV, due to the greater toxic potential of the drug when administered by this route. It is *doubtful* that *this route* of administration is *ever indicated* in acute myocardial infarction.

Dosage

1. Oral.
Quinidine preparations are available in 200 mg. tablets or capsules. Slow absorption preparations are also available.
   a. Quinidine dosage is related to body weight and must be given according to body size.[125,169]
   b. The dosage of quinidine depends also on kidney function. If the BUN is over 25 mg./100 ml. the plasma level of quinidine may be very high and toxicity may develop.

2. Intramuscular. Quinidine gluconate is the preparation used.

3. Intravenous (probably *not* indicated in acute myocardial infarction).
   a. Quinidine gluconate as a dilute solution in 5% glucose is infused slowly, with continuous observation of the patient and of the ECG. (0.8 Gm./250 ml.: Infuse at a maximum rate of 40 mg./minute.)
   b. IV injection should be undertaken only in hospitalized patients.
   c. The patient receiving quinidine therapy must be under close clinical observation. Continuous ECG and blood pressure observations are mandatory in order to detect any change in rate, rhythm or blood pressure. Administration of the drug must be stopped when any one of the following occurs:
      1) Side effects of more than a trivial nature.
      2) Restoration of sinus rhythm.
      3) Prolongation of QRS complex in excess of 25% beyond that observed before beginning of injection.
      4) Disappearance of P-waves.
      5) Decrease in heart rate to 120 beats/minute in tachyarrhythmias.

General Considerations

1. In therapeutic use the dosage of quinidine is variable and the effective dose must be determined for each patient.

2. In acute coronary care, quinidine may be useful for the purpose of suppressing auricular premature contractions, the dose being 0.2–0.3 Gm. every 6 hours. (*Note:* APCs frequently indicate heart failure, in which case digitalization will correct the APCs as atrial size decreases with cardiac compensation.)

3. It should be noted that the methods of scheduling the administration of quinidine vary, depending on the arrhythmia, the length of time the arrhythmia has been present and other factors in cardiac patients who do not have acute myocardial infarction.

4. Quinidine has not been sufficiently studied in acute coronary care for indications and appropriate dosage to be defined. Furthermore, due to the efficacy of lidocaine and procainamide, quinidine is not likely to receive extensive clinical investigation for acute coronary care use.

Toxic Effects

Toxicity due to Allergy

True allergic reactions, manifesting sensitization after prior exposure to the drug, are not common. These manifestations, however, are serious and are as follows:
1. Skin eruptions and angioneurotic edema.
2. Drug fever, sometimes with hyperpyrexia.
3. Asthma.
4. Serious episodes of thrombocytopenic purpura.
5. Hemolytic anemia.

Toxicity due to Idiosyncrasy

Intolerance via idiosyncrasy for relatively low doses of quinidine may be manifested by symptoms of either the gastrointestinal tract or the central nervous system and is far more common than allergic reactions. The manifestations of toxicity are as follows:
1. Gastrointestinal reactions.
   a. The commonest reason for discontinuance of quinidine therapy is the development of gastrointestinal symptoms, such as nausea, vomiting or diarrhea and abdominal cramps.
   b. Gastrointestinal symptoms occur with low quinidine dosages and, unlike digitalis-induced gastrointestinal symptoms, are *not* closely correlated with cardiovascular toxicity.
      1) 20–25% of patients experience gastrointestinal symptoms.
2. Central nervous system reactions.
   a. The most serious CNS complication due to quinidine therapy is central depression associated with respiratory arrest, convulsions and death. It has been demonstrated in animals that this syndrome can occur quite suddenly and at low dosage.

b. Susceptible patients most commonly develop, at low doses, visual and aural complaints of "cinchonism." These reactions preclude further use of quinidine, being absolute contraindications to the use of the drug.

Cardiovascular Toxicity

1. Decreased myocardial contractility and function is probably the most significant cardiovascular toxic effect.
   a. Doses in the "safe" therapeutic range probably do not significantly depress contractility in *normal* hearts. The "safe" dose for acutely injured hearts has not been determined.
2. The pharmacologic effect of prolonged conduction time (decreased conduction velocity) manifest by quinidine can cause severe toxic effects in cardiovascular response to quinidine overdose.
   a. The first clinical, apparent effects of quinidine are often ECG changes. These are:
      1) Prominence of the U wave.
      2) QT prolongation.
      3) QRS prolongation.
      4) PR interval increased.
      These manifestations do not properly represent toxicity but rather represent dose-related drug effects. At blood levels of 10 μg./ml. or higher, extreme cardiac toxicity with various transient arrhythmias which produce syncope or even sudden death are a dangerous possibility.
   b. Clinical experience has indicated that the degree of conduction prolongation as manifest by QRS prolongation correlates with cardiovascular toxicity.
      1) Prolonged QRS greater than 25–50% of the pretreatment QRS interval should preclude further increase in quinidine dosage.
3. With higher doses, SA block may result from depression of excitability and conduction.
4. Quinidine may cause unpredictable abnormalities of rhythm in digitalized hearts.
5. Hypotension is clearly a toxic effect. Hypotension due to toxic doses of quinidine is brought about by depression of cardiac contractility and reduction in peripheral resistance. Arterial blood pressure may be reduced to a serious degree with parenteral use of quinidine.

   a. Large oral doses of quinidine also normally reduce arterial blood pressure in man.
6. "Quinidine syncope" is caused by ventricular fibrillation at low doses.[270]

Treatment of Overdosages

1. To reduce the incidence and severity of allergic and idiosyncratic reactions, a quinidine test dose has long been recommended. This requirement further negates the likelihood of the use of quinidine as a primary drug in acute myocardial infarction.
2. Clinical experience with drugs in the treatment of quinidine intoxication in the cardiac patient is limited.
3. Most of the drugs commonly used in raising the blood pressure by increasing peripheral resistance are ineffective in the presence of quinidine intoxication.
   a. Apparently this is because of the quinidine-induced paralysis of arteriolar vasoconstriction.
   b. Arteriolar response to angiotensin (Hypertensin) is retained to some extent, and this drug also favorably affects heart rate and stroke volume. Thus, this naturally occurring polypeptide sympathomimetic agent is moderately effective in quinidine-induced hypotension.
   c. In animals, the effects of angiotensin have been potentiated by simultaneous administration of disodium calcium EDTA.
   d. The recent realization that the organic buffer THAM has some favorable effects suggests that correcting acidosis rather than increasing sodium is the specific mechanism of action, as THAM contains no sodium.
4. On the basis of the scanty information available, it would seem that administration of a titrated amount of intravenous angiotensin in molar sodium lactate or an equivalent amount of THAM, with subsequent titration of buffer as needed, is the best currently available treatment of quinidine toxicity.[99]
5. Sodium bicarbonate or sodium lactate may be used to treat quinidine toxicity.
6. Isoproterenol (Isuprel) is sometimes used in hypotension or AV block.
7. Direct-current electric shock is used for repeated episodes of ventricular fibrillation.

CHAPTER 10

Antiarrhythmic Therapeutic Procedures

Cardiac Pacing

TYPES OF PACING

There are several types of cardiac pacing currently employed. These are:[157]

1. Set rate (conventional) pacing.
2. *Demand pacing.*
3. Atrial synchronized pacing.
4. Paired pacing (paired atrioventricular pacing).
5. Coupled pacing.
   a. Atrial.
   b. Ventricular.

Types 1, 2 and 3 are most frequently utilized; the balance of the types are currently under more comprehensive study.

Pacing To Control Bradyarrhythmias

DISCUSSION

As the application of cardiac pacing in the brady-arrhythmias has not statistically significantly lowered the total over-all mortality rates for bradyarrhythmias in the presence of acute myocardial infarction, the justifiable question arises of whether or not the use of electrode catheters and cardiac pacemakers is of any value. It must be recalled, however, that many of the total number of bradyarrhythmias occur after onset of one of the types of mechanical heart failure (cardiogenic shock, pulmonary edema, congestive heart failure). Despite the uncertainties, many physicians who deal with heart block in the presence of acute myocardial infarction in large medical centers believe that electrode catheter insertion with pacemaking is sometimes lifesaving. The rationale for insertion of pacemaker electrodes and use of pacemakers in bradyarrhythmic disturbances is as follows:

1. For the avoidance of Adams-Stokes syndrome, which may be fatal.
2. For the prevention or alleviation of heart failure which may be due in part to slow cardiac rate and decreased cardiac output.

3. For possible reduction in the incidence of ventricular fibrillation to which slow rates predispose. Isoproterenol therapy for bradyarrhythmias, when used, particularly predisposes to ventricular fibrillation.
4. For the ability to use antiarrhythmic but cardiac depressant drugs which would otherwise be contraindicated.

On the other hand, an argument against the use of cardiac pacing in the bradyarrhythmias is that, even when complete AV block has been maintained, if there are no other serious complications, advanced heart block may not significantly alter the prognosis in infarction of the diaphragmatic myocardial wall.[151] This argument becomes invalid when we consider that:

1. Other complications *do frequently occur* in association with AV blocks of advanced degree.
2. Only slightly over 50% of the infarcts associated with advanced AV block are diaphragmatic infarcts.

It would appear that transvenous bipolar electrode catheter insertion and demand cardiac pacing definitely do have a place in the therapy of bradyarrhythmias associated with acute myocardial infarction.

Little benefit from pacing has been shown in patients suffering from severe infarction associated with shock, those resuscitated from cardiac arrest or those who have gross congestive failure.[64] However, in *less severely ill patients*, the mortality rate is considerably *improved* by use of cardiac pacing.[152] Therefore, there is a tendency to early insertion of pacing catheters for more positive control in this group of patients.

INDICATIONS FOR PACEMAKER THERAPY

1. Sinus node dysfunction with bradycardia.*
   a. An increasing number of authorities are inserting pacing catheters as a prophylactic measure at the time of initial appearance of bradycardia or for active cardiac pacing if drug therapy is unsuccessful. This early use is based on the increased

---

*References: 3, 21, 26, 34, 35, 63, 64, 87, 141.

awareness of the evolution of more advanced AV blocks from sinus bradycardia, and the finding that the mortality rate is considerably improved when pacing is utilized in the less severely ill patient.

b. Others[35,87] feel this is not necessary as an initial step and treat bradycardia by medical means.

c. Atrial pacing has been used in this situation.[26,63] If AV block supervenes, the pacing catheter is advanced into the right ventricle.

2. Normal sinus rhythm associated with the *emergence* of intraventricular conduction disturbances (left, right, bilateral or undefined bundle branch block).

a. It is generally agreed that this condition may provide an indication for insertion of a pacing electrode, and probably active pacing, as more advanced AV blocks usually follow.

3. First-degree AV block (prolonged PR interval).

a. If this is the sole manifestation of abnormal AV conduction, a pacemaker catheter is not inserted by most clinicians. If it represents an observed change in AV conduction, or if a change in conduction should follow a prolonged PR interval, a pacemaker electrode is frequently inserted for standby use.

4. Second-degree AV block.†

a. This situation usually just precedes complete heart block. Many authorities insert an electrode catheter and employ cardiac pacing in this situation if Mobitz type II block is present.

5. Third-degree (complete) AV block.‡

6. Slow nodal rhythm,[34,156] when medical therapy is not successful.

7. Episodes of cardiac arrest (asystole).[87]

8. Possibly inferior (diaphragmatic) infarction in the elderly,[34,35] particularly if there is a previous history of antecedent anterior myocardial infarction (i.e., multiple coronary artery disease involving the septal muscle and entire conduction system).

CONTROVERSIAL INDICATIONS FOR PACEMAKER THERAPY

1. Patients seen with complete AV block following an extensive myocardial infarction and presenting with *severe* cardiogenic shock, heart failure and unconsciousness—these patients have all died despite adequate pacing.[87]

a. In this particular group a more rapid and direct approach via transthoracic percutaneous pacing might be attempted.[87,142]

b. Often in patients with cardiogenic shock complete AV block suddenly develops (50–60% of patients with complete AV block and acute myocardial infarction seen in the coronary care unit),

†References: 15, 21, 26, 34, 35, 87, 140, 141, 174.
‡References: 15, 21, 26, 34, 35, 63, 76, 87, 140, 141, 174

with asystole occurring before a pacing electrode can be inserted.

c. This situation is also common in patients with pulmonary edema which responds poorly to treatment.

d. In these situations some authorities[26] insert a pacing electrode prophylactically in the more severely decompensated patients with acute myocardial infarction.

e. Unfortunately, in this general group with complications of "pump failure," few survive.

Pacing to Control Tachyarrhythmias and Myocardial Irritability

PATHOLOGIC PHYSIOLOGY

Just as there is a "critical rate" in patients who have complete heart block, there is also a "critical rate" in patients who do not have heart block, and by driving the heart above this rate (overdriving the heart) it is possible to wipe out multifocal ventricular ectopic activity. This ability is based solely on having the paced rate exceed the spontaneous rate and has nothing to do with the presence or absence of complete heart block.[155]

INDICATIONS IN TACHYARRHYTHMIAS WITH OR WITHOUT AV DISSOCIATION

1. Multiple ventricular ectopic beats[64,155,163] not controlled by medical therapy.
2. Recurrent ventricular tachycardia.[64,141,155,163]
3. Recurrent ventricular fibrillation.[64,155,163]
4. Supraventricular arrhythmias.
   a. Without drug therapy.
   b. In combination with drug therapy.[155]
   c. If supraventricular tachyarrhythmia is
      1) Not responsive to drugs;
      2) Pulmonary edema develops, or
      3) Shock occurs,
      atrial pacing is preferred. (See also Supraventricular Tachycardias in Chapter 4.)

PLACEMENT OF ELECTRODE

1. When AV conduction is intact, the pacing electrodes are placed in the atrium rather than the ventricle.[64,155]
   a. This avoids many of the risks associated with insertion of an electrode into the ventricle.
   b. It adds the beneficial effect of maintenance of atrial transport of conduction.
   c. By overdriving the heart from the atrium, a higher rate can be used than with ventricular pacing.
      1) This is beneficial in rapid rates due to the booster pump effect of atrial contraction.
      2) With slow heart rates there is little benefit in maintaining atrial systole.

2. When any degree of AV block is present, the electrode tip is placed in the right ventricle; or if AV block develops, the tip is advanced into the right ventricle.

The Process of Pacing

METHODS OF INSERTING ELECTRODE

Transvenous electrode pacing catheters may be inserted in any of the following ways:
1. In the cardiac catheterization laboratory, using image intensifier fluoroscopic control.
2. Percutaneous transvenously at the bedside, using the catheter tip as a unipolar intracavitary exploring ECG electrode, to determine the changing position of the electrode tip.
3. With the development of a portable image amplifier, catheter placement may be done in the coronary care unit under fluoroscopic control.

GENERAL TECHNIQUE

In *all* instances of electrode placement, a cardiac monitor, defibrillation equipment and artificial pulmonary ventilation equipment should be present.

Descriptions of electrode catheter insertion under fluoroscopic control, maneuvers to secure good myocardial wall contact, testing procedures and attachment of pacemaker generators are available in the literature.[21,34,35,64,76,163] An excellent discussion of pacemaker generators and their features is available.[64]

The "blind" method of insertion has been described.[29,146,218] Some consider the risks of "blind" positioning to be too high for the technique to be recommended and favor other methods of emergency management, such as IV administration of sympathomimetic amine or percutaneous chest wall needle placement of the pacing electrode.[163] It has been pointed out that the technique of "blind" placement is successful in only 65-72% of patients even in experienced hands.[63,218] In this method of electrode placement, the advancing tip of the pacing electrode is used as a unipolar exploring intracavitary lead for ECG determination of the position of the electrode tip.

The types of electrodes available include stiff pacing catheters, floating wires, "semi-floating" electrodes[218] and percutaneous transthoracic electrodes. Subcutaneous needles or plate electrodes in the chest wall were described in the early experience with electrode catheters and were used as the ground lead for unipolar electrode pacing catheters.

Transesophageal cardiac pacing as a temporary emergency method for cardiac pacing has been accomplished and recently described.[121] However, preliminary experiments with transesophageal electrodes in animals indicate that this would probably not be a practical method of driving the heart.[243]

The bipolar pacing electrode is always preferable and more reliable.

FACTORS COMMON TO ALL METHODS

1. Use sterile technique.
2. The question of which vein to use arises. Some feel the external jugular vein is preferable.[34,76] Others feel the antecubital, basilic or cephalic vein is preferable.[21,63] Still others have used the subclavian or saphenous vein.
   a. If an arm vein is used, the arm must be carefully splinted and the electrode itself placed without tension to prevent its movement from the endocardial wall, once properly placed.
3. The ECG and pulse are observed throughout the procedure and means for immediate defibrillation and pulmonary ventilation are available.
4. Positioning electrode catheter tip:
   a. The electrode tip is passed through the tricuspid valve and then into the pulmonary artery by some, thus demonstrating that it is not inadvertently placed into the coronary sinus. The tip is then withdrawn and maneuvered into position as low in the right ventricle and as far out in the apex as is possible.[21] The patient is then encouraged to breathe deeply, cough and turn on his side. If these maneuvers interrupt pacing, another position must be found for the electrode.
   b. Some investigators place the catheter tip into the main pulmonary artery fluoroscopically, and from this position withdraw it slowly into the midright ventricle, where pacing will be stable and the slight inevitable motion will not displace the electrode catheter. Others have found this method unsatisfactory due to the variable threshold of ventricular stimulation caused by the changing position of the electrode tip.
   c. If the electrode catheter tip is displaced into any of the following positions the pacemaker may not function properly, and stimulation may not occur.[76]
      i. Right atrium.
      ii. Pulmonary artery.
      iii. Too near the tricuspid valve—where displacement is easy and frequent.
      iv. It has also been suggested that, when the pacemaker electrode is in contact with the necrotic portion of the infarcted septum, the heart cannot be stimulated; and that when it is placed in the surrounding ischemic zone, which is hyperirritable, arrhythmias may be induced in the presence of AV block.[152]
   d. It may be necessary to try several positions before a stable pacing site is found.
   e. In the "blind" method of electrode insertion, the tip of the catheter electrode is used as an exploratory intracavitary lead to determine the position of the catheter tip.[63,155]
      i. The proximal tip of the electrode is connected to the V-lead terminal of the ECG.[155]

ii. A battery powered ECG is necessary to prevent possible 60-cycle current leakage to the injured heart.

PACEMAKER UNIT

1. Transvenous bipolar catheter electrodes with portable, battery operated demand pacemaker generators appear to be the preferred apparatus.[35]
   a. A reliable demand pacemaker avoids competitive rhythm.
   b. Battery operated units are preferred for internal stimulation in order to eliminate the possibility of ventricular fibrillation or pacing failure secondary to a leak of alternating 60-cycle current.
   c. The portable battery demand pacemaker may be shut off when sinus rhythm returns and withdrawn if sinus rhythm persists.
      1) Pacemakers, including demand type, should be OFF when sinus rhythm is present. The demand type has the advantage that there is less likelihood of competition at the time of re-establishment of normal sinus rhythm.
2. The demand type pacemaker does not remove all danger of ventricular fibrillation, and the underlying arrhythmia must be treated aggressively.[153]

THRESHOLD FOR PACING

1. After the pacemaker electrode is placed and the pacemaker attached, the threshold for stimulation must be determined.
   a. The threshold for pacing should be less than 1 ma., though some patients will require up to 2.5 ma. at threshold when the electrode tip is properly placed.[76] If more current is required, it can be assumed that the catheter tip is incorrectly positioned for optimal stimulation.
   b. After an optimal threshold is determined, the demand pacer impulse is generally set at 2 to 3 times threshold level to decrease the possibility of repetitive ventricular firing.[6,63]

COMPLICATIONS OF PACEMAKER THERAPY

The following are the complications which may occur during placement and/or use of the electrode catheter.

Occurring During Either Placement or Use

1. Malplacement of transvenous electrode. Function depends on the position of the tip of the electrode; placement and retention depend on the type of electrode and the skill of the operator.[64,76]
2. Perforation of the ventricle.[6,34,35,64,76] This rarely is a cause of cardiac tamponade.
3. Ventricular tachyarrhythmia during and following insertion of electrode catheter.[6,34,35]
   a. Due to irritation of myocardium during catheter passage.
   b. Due to stimulation of the injured myocardium during the vulnerable period.
      1. Most apt to occur with fixed rate pacemakers.

Occurring Only During Placement

1. Vein perforation.

Occurring Only During Pacemaker Use

1. Pacing failure, e.g., runaway pacemaker (must immediately disconnect or cut the electrode as a high mortality rate is associated with this situation if uncorrected).[34,35]
2. Competition[64] (unlikely with demand type pacemakers).
3. Exit block, i.e., increase of the excitation threshold above the capabilities of the pacemaker.[64]
4. Electrode fracture[64,76] (uncommon since use of coiled wire electrodes with better alloys).
5. Thrombophlebitis in cutdown vein.[34]
6. Local infection at site of cutdown.[34,76] One third of the patients will have this problem. Usually the infection will respond to local therapy.

Cardioversion

MECHANISM OF ACTION

Cardioversion has as its basic principle of action the depolarization of the entire heart. This total heart depolarization transiently extinguishes all electrical activity and permits the opportunity for the sinus node to resume as the dominant cardiac pacemaker.

INDICATIONS

General reasons for cardioversion in the presence of acute myocardial infarction are:
1. To control heart rate.
2. To return the effect of atrial systole followed by ventricular systole for more efficient pumping action.
3. Cardioversion is instituted when one or both of the foregoing conditions are not controllable by drugs, or when the urgency of the situation does not permit institution of drug therapy.

Specific indications for cardioversion include:
1. Any tachycardia, except sinus tachycardia, when shock and/or pulmonary edema are present.
   a. Contraindication: digitalis-induced tachycardia.
2. Supraventricular tachycardia, when the heart rate does not slow adequately with digitalis therapy, or when rapid development of pulmonary edema does not permit time to administer digitalis.

a. Use caution with cardioversion in the presence of digitalis or digitalis toxicity.
3. If auricular fibrillation or flutter of the following types exist:
   a. Of recent onset via acute myocardial infarction, with rate not controlled by digitalis and failure developing.
   b. With rapid development of pulmonary edema, not allowing time for digitalis therapy.
      1) Contraindication: if auricular fibrillation or flutter is associated with:
         a) Digitalis toxicity.
         b) Is drug induced, or
         c) If advanced degrees of AV block are present.
4. Nodal tachycardia, not responding to medical measures or with heart failure.
   a. Contraindication: digitalis-induced tachycardia.
5. Ventricular tachycardia, when the following conditions exist:
   a. Decreased cardiac output is occurring, manifest as rapid severe development of shock or pulmonary edema. (See Ventricular Tachycardia, groups II and III for purposes of therapy, in Chapter 4.)
6. Ventricular fibrillation.
   a. Cardioversion defibrillation may be effective in temporarily terminating ventricular tachycardia or fibrillation in about 90% of cases if delivered rapidly after onset.
7. Asystole.
   a. Sudden asystole.
   b. Asystole following AV block.

CONTRAINDICATION (DIGITALIS INTOXICATION)

In general, cardioversion is contraindicated in arrhythmias due to digitalis toxicity.[263,264] If the arrhythmia itself is progressing toward an obvious, rapid termination of the patient's life, it might be necessary to try cardioversion as a primary treatment. However, attempts to *premedicate* with antiarrhythmic agents should be made in order to protect from the ventricular fibrillation that can occur with cardioversion in the face of digitalis toxicity, and to increase the possibility that the cardioversion will be effective once the countershock is delivered. The agents which have been utilized are:
1. Lidocaine. Many feel this to be the drug of choice.
2. Diphenylhydantoin (Dilantin).
3. Propranolol (Inderal).

It is preferable to treat arrhythmias that occur with digitalis toxicity by medical means if at all possible (i.e., if the arrhythmia is not immediately life threatening).

Technique of Cardioversion

PREMEDICATION WITH ANTIARRHYTHMIC AGENTS

Antiarrhythmic agents are administered to avoid the development of severe ventricular arrhythmias, if urgency of the situation does not prevent this premedication.
1. The premedication will frequently have been accomplished as part of the therapy of the arrhythmia prior to a decision to cardiovert.
2. In the event of ventricular tachycardia, with decreased cardiac output and rapid heart failure or asystole, *immediate* cardioversion is indicated.
   a. Initiate lidocaine therapy as soon as possible.
3. In the event of ventricular fibrillation, *immediate* defibrillation is indicated.
4. Drugs used as antiarrhythmic premedication before cardioversion are:
   a. Lidocaine, 1–2 mg./kg. as an IV bolus, followed by infusion of 1–2 mg./minute is probably the drug of choice on the basis of experience to date.
   b. Diphenylhydantoin 100–250 mg. given IV over 4–5 minutes.
      1) *Caution:* Give slowly, as cardiac arrests have been precipitated by rapid IV doses of this drug.
   c. Propranolol, 1–3 mg. IV, has been used in refractory ventricular arrhythmias prior to cardioversion.

PREMEDICATION WITH ANESTHETIC AGENTS

In the conscious patient, the following dosages are used.
1. Valium, 5 mg. IV every 5 minutes, to a total dose of 20 mg.[154]
2. Valium, in doses of 10–20 mg. IV given in 60–90 seconds.[73]
   a. Valium has not been associated with VPCs as has thiopental sodium.[73]
3. Thiopental sodium has been used in the operating room[154] or the coronary care unit[22,73] as a 1% solution, 250–400 mg. usually being given.

METHODS OF PADDLE PLACEMENT

The paddle electrodes of the defibrillator have been placed by various authorities as follows:
1. At the level of the fourth to fifth interspace, one to the right of the sternum and the other horizontally to the left in the anterior axillary line.
2. In an oblique position, with one paddle to the right of the sternum at the second interspace and one to the left at the fourth to fifth interspace at the anterior axillary line. This is probably the most commonly used positioning.
3. One electrode placed posteriorly and one anteriorly.

ELECTRICAL CHARGE

1. Skin must be dry, electrodes clean and shiny and

the electrode paste well spread. Paste-electrode-skin contact must be good to avoid loss of energy and resultant low-energy charge.

2. Synchronized charge delivered during the *non-vulnerable* phase is preferable if there is time. When time is of the essence in ventricular arrhythmias, do not hesitate to deliver nonsynchronized charge.
   a. Synchronized charge is delivered on the downstroke of the R-wave or, if a good R-wave is not present, on the upstroke of the S-wave.
   b. If the charge is not synchronized, ventricular fibrillation may occur.
3. Larger shocks for ventricular fibrillation avoid the partial depolarization and resultant predisposition to continued ventricular fibrillation that may occur with smaller shocks when ventricular fibrillation is present with acute myocardial infarction.
   a. High-energy shock levels are frequently used

initially in order to terminate the arrhythmia as rapidly as possible.
   1) DC shock is generally preferred.
   b. Deliver DC shock of 200–400 watt-seconds, and repeat several times if necessary.
   c. If ineffective, attempts are made to make the myocardium more responsive by giving sodium bicarbonate, epinephrine and calcium while cardiopulmonary resuscitation is being carried out; then cardioversion is again attempted.
4. For supraventricular arrhythmias and ventricular tachycardia a smaller charge of 50 watt-seconds, followed by 100, 200 and 400 watt-seconds, respectively, should be administered when there is time, as larger charges, in these situations, tend to produce ventricular irritability.
   a. *Premedicate* with an antiarrhythmic agent (lidocaine).

Cardiopulmonary Resuscitation—Cardiac Arrest[§]

DISCUSSION

In discussing cardiac arrest and cardiopulmonary resuscitation it must be noted that the divisions artificially made to discuss the subject do not actually exist, but are merely a convenience for presentation of the material. Definitive therapy must be started as soon as possible after initiation of the other measures of cardiopulmonary resuscitation. In this discussion it must also be remembered that we are considering a patient who is being monitored electrocardiographically in an intensive coronary care unit, and not a patient at large in the hospital.

The term "cardiac arrest" conveys, on first glance, the meaning of cardiac asystole. Actually few instances of cardiac arrest are primarily due to the occurrence of cardiac asystole. "Cardiac arrest" then is defined as the sudden failure of the heart to maintain adequate circulation, resulting in inadequate oxygenation of the vital organs of the body, in particular the brain. Cardiopulmonary resuscitation is carried out so that the brain may survive until an adequate diagnosis and definitive therapy of the underlying cause may be undertaken. In acute myocardial infarction the cause of cardiac arrest is nearly always an arrhythmia.

The object of cardiopulmonary resuscitation is to maintain the vital functions after *clinical death,* so that *biologic death* does not occur. Clinical death is said to be present when no audible heart beat, palpable pulse or breathing can be detected. Biologic death occurs when cellular anoxia and anaerobic glycolysis have proceeded to a state of irreversible deterioration in the brain. Brain death is represented by a linear ("flat") EEG recording. When clinical death occurs, it is recognized by absent pulse, apnea and dilatation of pupils.

The pupils begin to dilate within 30–45 seconds following cerebral anoxia. In the acute coronary care unit, the presence of an arrhythmia heralding the onset of clinical death will be observed almost instantaneously, and action can be taken quickly. Within 4–6 minutes (probably only 4 minutes) after the onset of clinical death, the cerebral cortex suffers irreparable damage.

Just as the pupils begin to dilate quickly after clinical death, with the institution of effective ventilation and circulation they begin to constrict quickly. Thus the pupils are a convenient indicator for progress of resuscitation and prognosis.

A determination of whether cardiopulmonary resuscitation should be undertaken depends on the patient's being reached before biologic death and being salvageable. The sudden onset of cardiac arrest in a patient with a "good heart" is most certainly an indication to institute cardiopulmonary resuscitation.

The incidence of cardiac arrest and the survival rate in coronary care units have been drastically changed due to the early treatment of cardiac arrhythmias.

The vital functions which must be restored and maintained during cardiopulmonary resuscitation are the (1) cardiac, (2) circulatory, (3) ventilatory and (4) metabolic functions.

General Procedures in Counteracting Clinical Death

The general steps of cardiopulmonary resuscitation are the A-B-C-D of therapy for cardiac arrest and institution of cardiopulmonary resuscitation:
Airway.
Breathing.
Circulation.
Definitive therapy.

[§]References: 33, 36, 107, 219, 220, 223, 240.

GENERAL THERAPY

Following are some of the general steps and general information applicable to cardiopulmonary resuscitation. The A-B-C-D of resuscitation will be taken up individually in the next section.

1. Expired air ventilation (mouth-to-mouth) is usually used.
   a. Oxygenation is more desirable, and an oxygen-filled bag is superior to expired air and should be used whenever possible.
2. External cardiac compression (manual cardiac massage) is initially used. If cardiac massage is to be continued, some centers are equipped with oxygen pressure-activated respiration-synchronized cardiac compression apparatus.
3. An initial dose of cardiotonic drug is indicated within the first 2 minutes of resuscitation.
   a. The IV route will usually have been secured on admission to the coronary care unit; if not, a venous cutdown will be necessary.
   b. Epinephrine is usually used and/or calcium chloride or gluconate (calcium ion).
4. Antacid solutions should be given initially and repeated at 8–10 minute intervals to combat metabolic acidosis.
   a. Sodium bicarbonate, 40–44.6 mEq. or 75 ml. of 5% solution, should be administered IV every 8–10 minutes.
   b. THAM may be utilized.
   c. Sodium lactate has been utilized.
5. Electrocardiographic evaluation must be undertaken as early as possible in resuscitation.
   a. In the coronary care unit, monitoring of ECG with rapid diagnosis of arrhythmia and early definitive therapy is possible.
   b. Ventricular tachycardia and ventricular fibrillation are the commonest causes of cardiac arrest. Defibrillate immediately. If it is possible to defibrillate within the first 30–60 seconds, defibrillate before instituting cardiopulmonary resuscitation.
   c. Advanced heart block, bradycardia and/or asystole are the other possible causes. Treat with electrode pacing (possibly transthoracic percutaneous electrode) and/or medical means while carrying out cardiopulmonary resuscitation.
6. Postresuscitative management involves maintenance of adequate ventilation, therapy of metabolic imbalances and prophylaxis to prevent return of arrhythmias.

Specific Steps (A-B-C-D) in Cardiopulmonary Resuscitation

A. MANAGEMENT OF AIRWAY

1. Tilt head back, one hand under neck, one hand on forehead.
2. Lift up jaws.

   a. Either one or both these maneuvers may open airway by bringing the tongue off the posterior pharynx.
3. Remove dentures and remove any food or foreign bodies from the mouth. (Suction if necessary.)
4. After airway control, start ventilation of the lungs.

B. VENTILATION (BREATHING)

Mouth-to-mouth is instantly available. Mouth-to-nose, mouth-to-S-tube, bag and mask may be used.

1. Institute lung inflation with oxygen and bag as soon as practical. (Inflate lungs 12 times/minute.)
2. An artificial airway and proper-fitting mask may be needed to facilitate airway control. Tracheal intubation is recommended to minimize aspiration when it can be done without loss of time and control.
   a. DO NOT delay initial oxygenation or mouth-to-mouth resuscitation for intubation.
3. Gastric decompression may be needed because of air in the stomach from ventilation efforts.
4. Emergency tracheostomy for laryngeal obstruction is seldom necessary in the coronary care unit.

C. ARTIFICIAL CIRCULATION (EXTERNAL CARDIAC MASSAGE)

1. The technique must be learned in an appropriate training course.
   a. Cardiac compression must be carried out 60 times/minute.
      1) Lungs inflated every fifth cardiac compression.
2. Even in the presence of efficient external cardiac massage, carotid artery flow is approximately 30–50% of normal.
3. Mechanism of action of external cardiac compression.
   a. During cardiac compression, blood is forced from the ventricles into the systemic and pulmonary circulation.
   b. Relaxation of the pressure permits the chest wall to recoil, causing relatively negative pressure and flow of venous blood back into the atria and ventricles from the pulmonary and systemic circulation.
4. Some complications of closed chest cardiac massage are:
   a. Postmassage pulmonary edema.
   b. Fat or bone marrow emboli.
   c. Pneumothorax.
   d. Fracture of ribs, sternum, scapula, flail chest, costochondral separation.
   e. Hemothorax.
   f. Perforated viscus, ruptured spleen, hepatic laceration.
   g. Pericardial or myocardial laceration.
   h. *Permanent brain damage.*

D. DEFINITIVE THERAPY

Ideally, much of the definitive therapy is undertaken while the A-B-Cs of cardiopulmonary resuscitation are taking place. Procedures and therapy which are considered definitive therapy are:

1. Securing an IV route for medications if one is not available.
2. Treating metabolic acidosis, which occurs within 5 minutes after cardiac arrest even with adequate cardiopulmonary resuscitation. Therapy consists of sodium bicarbonate, 50 ml. ampule of 44.6 mEq. or 75 ml. of 5% solution administered IV every 8–10 minutes.
3. Treating hypotension via IV infusion of Levophed or Aramine.
   a. Levophed (levarterenol bitartrate), 16 mg. in 500 ml. of 5% D/W.
   b. Aramine (metaraminol), 200 mg. in 500 ml. of 5% D/W.
   c. Hydrocortisone (Solu-Cortef) may be given IV, if vasopressors are ineffective.
4. Endotracheal intubation with cuffed tube to simplify airway and minimize aspiration. Maintain ventilation manually or by mechanical respirator.
5. Increasing myocardial strength and irritability for defibrillation (if arrest is due to ventricular tachycardia or ventricular arrhythmia). Initially adminster 0.5 mg. epinephrine by intracardiac injection, cutdown or IV (dilute 1 mg. to 10 ml. and give 5 ml. of this at one time).
6. Restoring spontaneous, effective cardiac activity.
   a. Obtain ECG immediately: usually attached to monitor in coronary care unit.
   b. If ventricular fibrillation is present:
      1) Defibrillate immediately.
      2) If fibrillation is of low amplitude, convert to coarse fibrillation by intracardiac injection of 0.5 mg. epinephrine (5 ml. of 1:10,000 solution).
      3) If weak fibrillation persists, inject 10% calcium chloride—5 ml. to achieve coarse fibrillation.
      4) Defibrillate at 400 watt-seconds initially in this circumstance.
      5) If ventricular fibrillation persists, external cardiac compression and ventilation are resumed.
         a) Procainamide (200 mg. IV) or lidocaine (50 mg. IV or intracardiac) may be necessary before repeating countershock.
   c. In ventricular asystole, slow idioventricular rhythm or extreme sinus bradycardia:
      1) Pacemaker must be used (possibly percutaneous transthoracic). Pace at rate of 70–80/minute at whatever power level is required for cardiac stimulation.
         a) External cardiac pacemaker is usually ineffective in this circumstance.
      2) Isoproterenol (Isuprel) may be effective in initiating or enhancing cardiac rhythmicity. Give IV in dose of 0.02–0.1 mg. every 3–5 minutes. Maintenance therapy by IV infusion (2 mg. per 500 ml. of 5% D/W).
      3) Atropine has also been given for AV block.
7. Watching for indications of irreversible brain damage. Resuscitation is considered unsuccessful if the pupils remain dilated and nonreactive and no spontaneous respiration or ECG activity occurs for more than an hour. (Various times have been suggested.)
8. Keeping of some sort of flow chart by supervisory nursing personnel. Preferably this should be based on the time from an elapsed timer. Most institutions design a chart particularly fitted to their needs and subsequent study procedures. A simple flow chart has been published in the literature.[36] (See also Appendix.)

Postresuscitation Care[33,107]

1. Intensive postresuscitation therapy will usually be necessary for 72–96 hours.
2. Support ventilation. Respiratory alkalosis with concomitant fall in serum potassium level may occur with artificial ventilation.
3. Minimize cerebral edema via osmotic diuretics (mannitol) or hypothermia.
4. Monitor urine production with an indwelling catheter in the bladder. Flow should be maintained at above 30 ml./hour.
5. Support blood pressure via vasopressors and cardiotonic drugs.
6. Observe for and control metabolic acidosis or other electrolyte imbalance.
   a. In patients with previous pulmonary problems, respiratory acidosis is prevalent.
   b. If there was no previous pulmonary problem, metabolic acidosis is the usual finding.[220]
   c. Ideally, facilities for analyzing blood gases and pH should be available.

PROTOCOL

A representative protocol of recommended steps for cardiopulmonary resuscitation for nurse and physician is available in the Appendix of this manual.

Anticoagulation Therapy*

INDICATIONS

There is no complete agreement concerning the indications for anticoagulation therapy or the length of time it should be continued as long-term therapy in coronary artery disease with or without acute myocardial infarction. Many clinicians feel that short-term anticoagulant therapy should be carried out for at least several weeks in the presence of acute myocardial infarction, provided no contraindication to anticoagulation exists. The purpose of anticoagulation therapy has been established to be the significant reduction of thromboembolic complications; anticoagulant therapy does not affect the other major causes of death in acute myocardial infarction.[250]

It is especially agreed that poor-risk patients should receive anticoagulant therapy. These poor-risk patients include those with:
1. Previous infarction.
2. Intractable pain.
3. Shock.
4. Marked cardiac enlargement.
5. Heart failure.
6. Arrhythmias.
7. Other complicating diseases predisposing to coronary artery disease.

CONTRAINDICATIONS

Strict contraindications to anticoagulation therapy are:
1. A hemorrhagic diathesis.
2. Severe hypertension (diastolic pressure greater than 110–115 mm. Hg).
3. Active ulceration.
4. Overt bleeding from any site, including:
   a. Intracranial.
   b. Gastrointestinal.
   c. Genitourinary.
   d. Pulmonary (except for hemoptysis due to pulmonary emoblism).
5. Inadequate laboratory facilities.

6. Inadequate patient cooperation–not likely in acute coronary care.
7. Surgery of central nervous system.
8. Pregnancy (coumarin derivatives pass placental barrier, heparin does not).
9. Septal perforation.
10. Known hypersensitivity to the anticoagulant drugs.

Less stringent contraindications are:
1. Moderate hypertension.
2. Diabetes.
3. Vasculitis.
4. Renal and liver disease.
5. Surgery in general, but particularly surgery of the:
   a. Prostate.
   b. Lung.
   c. Biliary tract in the presence of hepatic failure.
6. Pericarditis complicating acute myocardial infarction. See Chapter 7.

METHOD OF ANTICOAGULATION

Anticoagulation, as usually carried out, begins with heparin for rapid anticoagulant effect and utilizes coumarin derivatives for slower onset but longer-lasting anticoagulation effect. A schema of the normal clotting mechanism may be seen in Figure 12.

Heparin

Heparin is a potent organic acid, which occurs naturally in the body in small amounts. It is a mixture of sulfate-containing mucopolysaccharides, with molecular weights ranging from 8,000 to 15,000. Its high content of ester sulfates gives heparin the highest negative electrical charge of any substance that can be safely injected into man. Heparin combines with a wide variety of proteins being bound to the amino groups to form sulfaminic linkages. Heparin also has pharmacologic effects other than anticoagulation.

Heparin is believed by many to be the anticoagulant

---

*References: 1, 7, 9, 10, 15, 25, 64, 90, 164, 191.

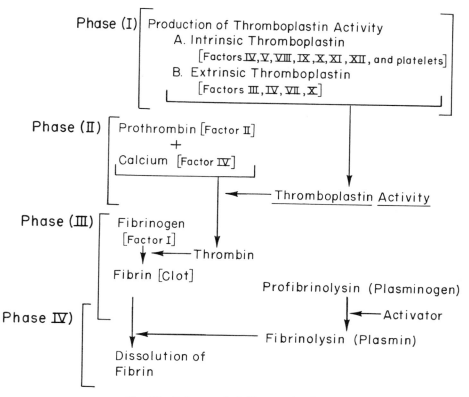

Fig. 12.—Schema of clotting mechanism.

of choice, but because of its cost and the necessity for parenteral administration, it is not practical for long-term administration. It is usually used in those patients with acute situations requiring immediate anti-coagulation.

ANTICOAGULANT ACTION

Heparin is a direct-acting anticoagulant. Its action is a direct result and reflection of its chemical properties. It is immediately effective. The drug acts on major components of the coagulation system:
1. On Phase I (see schema).
   a. It inhibits certain interactions involved in thromboplastin elaboration and prevents the activation of clotting factor IX.
2. On Phase II.
   a. In conjunction with a plasma cofactor, it inhibits the action of thrombin. Also, thrombin-induced aggregation of platelets may be prevented at high concentrations of heparin.
3. On Phase III.
   a. Thrombin-mediated conversion of fibrinogen to fibrin is retarded as an indirect result of thrombin action inhibition.
4. On Phase IV.
   a. There are *no* significant clinical effects on the fibrinolytic system.

OTHER ACTIONS

1. Heparin does not cross the placental barrier or appear in the milk, making it the preferred anticoagulant during pregnancy.
2. It activates endogenous lipoprotein lipase, causing "clearing" of postprandial lipemic serum.
3. There is interference with reactions involving complement and antigen-antibody interaction.
4. Heparin depresses aldosterone production.
5. It causes transient depression of platelet count.

METABOLISM

The exact routes of elimination of exogenously administered heparin are not precisely known. About 20% can be recovered in the urine. The rest is apparently detoxified in the liver by enzymes.

INDICATIONS AND CONTRAINDICATIONS FOR USE

Heparin therapy is prophylactic. Heparin's effect is *hopefully* to prevent distal propagation of the thrombus and to limit thrombin-mediated platelet accretion on the surface of the thrombus. The primary indication for heparin is the need to prevent new thrombus formation and thus thromboembolic episodes, particularly in the poor-risk patient.

Contraindications include any bleeding tendency, a hypersensitivity to heparin itself, which is rare, and other contraindications as enumerated under contraindications to anticoagulation therapy.

DOSAGE AND ADMINISTRATION

Heparin must be administered parenterally. It may be administered subcutaneously IV or IM. Intramuscular injections should be avoided because they are frequently associated with considerable bleeding into the injection site. Depoheparin is not generally recommended because of irregularity of absorption and frequent hematoma at the injection site. Heparin is not absorbed through buccal or rectal mucosa.

IV Administration

1. Aqueous sodium heparin is the preparation of choice.
2. There is no uniformity of opinion concerning the optimal dose of heparin, the frequency of administration or the method of regulating the dose.
3. Suggested dosage schedules are:
   a. 5,000–10,000 units IV every 4 hours, the dosage being controlled by clotting times. The dosage should be sufficient to maintain the whole blood clotting time 2–3 times the control value (Lee-White method) 3–4 hours after the last dose.
      1) This allows for changing anticoagulant effects and variations in heparin requirements.
      2) Patients sometimes require more heparin during the first 24–48 hours than they will require later.
   b. Others suggest that during the initial 48 hours of therapy, larger doses (10,000–15,000 units) be given IV at 4-hour intervals without regard to whole blood clotting times.

Other Routes of Administration

1. 15,000–20,000 units subcutaneously every 12 hours.
2. 5,000–10,000 units IV and 7,500 units subcutaneously every 6–8 hours, each subsequent dose dependent on clotting time.

TOXICITY (SHORT-TERM USE)

1. Essentially nontoxic in short-term treatment except for the hazard of hemorrhage.
2. Hypersensitivity.
3. The importance of pre-existent liver and renal damage must be evaluated in determining dosage.
4. The anticoagulant action is proportional to the dose. This action varies from patient to patient, and the effect becomes evident immediately after IV administration.
5. The guide to heparin dosage is the whole blood clotting time performed by the Lee-White method.

ANTIDOTE

The specific antidote to heparin is protamine sulfate. Protamines are simple proteins of low molecular weight that are rich in arginine and strongly basic. Protamine has a strong electrostatic affinity for heparin and combines with it to form a salt devoid of anticoagulant activity. Protamine alone has an anticoagulant effect, thus a dose as nearly precise as possible must be used to neutralize heparin. A useful schedule for neutralizing an IV dose of heparin is to administer 1 mg. protamine for every 100 units of heparin given at the last injection, noting that *an excess of protamine may prolong clotting*. This is done by diluting 5 ml. of a 1% solution of protamine to 25 ml. with isotonic saline and giving the appropriate amount, but not in excess of 100 mg. protamine. Protamine should be administered IV over 3–5 minutes to diminish the likelihood of reactions to the drug, such as sudden hypotension, bradycardia, dyspnea, transitory flushing and a feeling of warmth.

Neutralization of subcutaneous injections of heparin must be carried out with smaller doses of protamine given at intervals, because of the slower absorption of subcutaneously injected heparin.

Coumarin Derivatives

Bishydroxycoumarin and warfarin are the safest and most widely used preparations and are the only ones which will be considered here. The coumarin preparations vary individually in solubility and onset and length of action. The coumarin agents do traverse the placenta and are found in mothers' milk.

TOTAL ACTION

The coumarins act only in the liver. They retard the synthesis of certain procoagulants. Coumarin type compounds act by:
1. Inhibition of synthesis of intrinsic and extrinsic factors VII, IX and X in Phase I of the clotting mechanism, affecting thromboplastin activity.
2. Inhibition of synthesis of prothrombin (factor II) in Phase II of the clotting mechanism.

Special factors modify the activity of coumarin type anticoagulants[1,7,9,10,25,90] (other factors are being rapidly discovered):
1. Factors which *potentiate* the action of coumarin derivatives.
   a. Any factor which lowers the intake of vitamin K.
      1) Decrease in dietary fat.
      2) Antibiotic therapy—by suppression of normal intestinal flora which are important for the synthesis of vitamin K.
      3) Liver or kidney damage.
      4) Nonspecific factors—fever and stress.

b. Drugs which may displace coumarins from protein-binding sites in the plasma.
1) Phenbutazone.
2) Indomethacin.
3) Diphenylhydantoin.
4) Chloral hydrate.
c. Drugs which depress prothrombin formation in
the liver.
1) Salicylates in large doses.
2) Broad-spectrum antibiotics.
3) ACTH.
4) Corticosteroids.
5) Quinine, quinidine.
6) Clofibrate (Atromid-S).
7) Methylthiouracil.
8) Dextrothyroxine.
9) Norethindrone.
10) Some radioactive compounds.
2. Factors and drugs which *antagonize* the action of
coumarin type anticoagulants.
a. By stimulating metabolic degradation of the drug.
1) Griseofulvin.
2) Alcohol.
3) Barbiturates within 5 hours of ingestion of anticoagulant tablet.
4) Glutethimide (Doriden).
5) Meprobamate.
b. In other ways.
1) Vitamin K.
2) Neomycin.
3) Gastrointestinal disturbances with diarrhea.

METABOLISM

The coumarins are almost entirely bound to plasma
protein, probably albumin; about 99% are bound in
therapeutic dosage ranges. The drugs are present in
erythrocytes and in many organs. Coumarins are detoxified by the liver and disappear slowly from the
blood stream due to plasma binding.

INDICATIONS AND CONTRAINDICATIONS

See indications for heparin and for anticoagulation
therapy.

Hypersensitivity and bleeding with therapy are contraindications, as are drug and other interactions previously presented.

TOXICITY

Toxic effects other than hemorrhage are rarely seen.
(See also the special factors modifying activity under
Total Action.)

Reactions to all the coumarins are rare, and Dicumarol is the least toxic. Reactions which can occur
include nausea, vomiting, diarrhea, fever, jaundice,
leukopenia, thrombocytopenia, leukemoid reaction
and vasculitis.

LABORATORY CONTROL

In acute coronary care, determination of daily prothrombin times (Quick's one-step method) is advisable,
with adjustment of dosage accordingly. Heparin may
also affect the results of this laboratory test.

THERAPY WITH COUMARIN DERIVATIVES

1. Bishydroxycoumarin (Dicumarol) is available for oral
administration only. Usually 300 mg. is given the
first day, 200 mg. the second and 25–100 mg. the
third day and thereafter. Maintenance dose is variable. Anticoagulation is usually achieved in 2–3 days.
2. Warfarin (Coumadin, panwarfin) is available for
parenteral and oral use. 1 mg./kg. body weight, up
to 40–50 mg., is usually given the first day; none is
given the second day; dosage the third day and thereafter is dependent on prothrombin time. Maintenance
dose varies from 1 to 15 mg. daily, usually in range
of 5–10 mg. Anticoagulation effect is usually achieved
in 12–36 hours.

ANTIDOTE

Vitamin K_1 is the drug of choice. Vitamin K_1 may
be given orally, and water emulsions of vitamin K_1 are
available for parenteral use (Aquamephyton, mona-Kay,
Kanakion).

When parenteral administration is required, the IM
route is usually used. In those rare situations in which
IV administration is necessary, injections should be
slow (over 5–10 minutes) to avoid side reactions.

Therapy of Overdose

1. Prolonged prothrombin time but without bleeding:
Requires no treatment, omit 1 or 2 daily doses.
2. Prolonged prothrombin time with mild bleeding:
Oral administration of 5–10 mg. vitamin K_1.
3. Moderate bleeding: 10–20 mg. vitamin K_1 is given
IM. If bleeding is severe, 10–25 mg. may be given
IV slowly. Safe prothrombin times are often achieved
in 4–8 hours.
4. Bleeding without prolonged prothrombin time: 5–10
mg. vitamin K_1 orally.
5. Transfusion: Whole blood or plasma quickly antag-
onizes the effects of excess coumarin.
6. If bleeding occurs in what appears to be safe prothrombin time ranges, look for laboratory error or
some underlying organic lesion.

CHAPTER 12

Digitalis

In the discussion that follows the term "digitalis" will be used to designate the entire group of cardiac glycosides rather than to designate digitalis alone. The terms "digitalis," "digitalis preparations" and "cardiac glycosides" are used synonymously to include all the preparations of digitalis.

Digitalis preparations currently used are derived from plant sources. All the digitalis preparations are derived from the plant leaf, except ouabain which is derived from the plant seed. Some of the digitalis preparations are semisynthetic glycosides in that they are derived by esterification of the original glycosides.

All the cardiac glycosides produce qualitatively the same basic type of cardiac effect. There are, of course, quantitative differences in the actions of the various derivatives.

Action and Metabolism (Pharmacophysiology)

Mechanisms of Cardiovascular Action*

1. Increase in the force of myocardial contraction. This action is the main pharmacodynamic property of cardiac glycosides.
   a. Cardiac glycosides have been shown to increase the force of the nonfailing heart as well as to lower the oxygen debt of the nonfailing human heart.[88]
   b. Digitalis causes no significant hemodynamic changes in normal individuals, even with increased force of contraction.
2. Increase in cardiac output in the failing heart as a result of increased myocardial contractile force.
   a. Lowers elevated ventricular and diastolic pressures.
3. Cardiac glycosides affect electrical impulse conduction of the heart. *Therapeutic* doses produce the following effects on excitability and rhythmicity.
   a. Insignificant slowing of the heart rate via digitalis drug itself.
      1) In toxic doses the SA node is directly affected and there is also an increase in vagal tone, causing bradycardia.
      2) In therapeutic doses, in the presence of heart failure, the ventricular rate frequently slows because the heart failure is relieved by the cardiac glycoside.

   b. Conduction of the excitatory impulse through the atrium to the ventricles is slowed.
      1) This is manifest by an increased PR interval seen on the electrocardiogram and occurs via the direct action of digitalis on the conduction tissue.
   c. There are effects on the refractory period of the heart.
      1) Effective refractory period of the atrium is decreased.
      2) Effective refractory period of the AV node is increased by direct effects and reflex vagal effects.
      3) Refractory period of the ventricles is decreased.
         a) The decreased refractory period of the ventricles accompanied by the increased excitability of the ventricle may result in ventricular premature complexes, an important forewarning of more severe digitalis-induced ectopic ventricular arrhythmias (i.e., ventricular tachycardia and fibrillation).
   d. Slowing of the AV conduction.
      1) Toxic doses of digitalis slow conduction of impulses within the AV node, causing partial or complete heart block.

Biochemical Mechanisms of Action

1. Whatever the mechanism of action, digitalis glycosides appear to restore the utilization of energy by the

---

*References: 7, 10, 14, 15, 19, 38, 39, 72, 77, 94, 167, 231, 263, 264.

failing myocardium. There is an increased efficiency in conversion of metabolic to mechanical energy after digitalis administration which is reflected by an increase in cardiac oxygen consumption.

2. The exact mechanism of action of digitalis at the cellular level has not yet been determined with complete accuracy. The following discussion of the inotropic effect of digitalis is fragmentary at best and does not intermesh to produce a logical answer to the biochemical action of digitalis. The discussion is presented for informational purposes only. The inotropic effect of digitalis has been attributed to one or more of the following:

a. Influence on actin and actomyosin. There is evidence to suggest, but by no means conclusively prove, that the effect of cardiac glycosides is to increase contractility of bonds of actomyosin in the failing heart.

b. Action on the ATPase enzyme system.
   1) There is a correlation between the toxicity of various cardiac glycosides and their ability to inhibit cardiac ATPase.
   2) ATPase supplies energy for the sodium–potassium transport system.
   3) ATPase requires magnesium ion for activation and is inhibited by calcium.
      a) High concentrations of calcium inhibit the positive inotropic action of digitalis and potentiate the toxic effects.
      b) Magnesium transiently opposes signs of digitalis toxicity. Magnesium is necessary for activation of the sodium ion, potassium ion and ATPase interaction.

c. Modification of ion transport system across the myocardial cell membrane.
   1) Digitalis blocks the active transport of ions across cell membranes of a variety of tissues. Cardiac glycosides inhibit active transport of sodium and potassium ions in red blood cells. In the heart, potassium transfer from the extracellular space to the intracellular space is inhibited by digitalis.
      a) Increasing doses of digitalis cause potassium ion loss from the heart simultaneously with an improvement in contractility.
      b) High potassium concentrations protect the enzyme ATPase against inhibition by the glycosides and also protect against digitalis toxicity.

d. Stimulation of carbohydrate metabolism.

These possible mechanisms of digitalis action are not necessarily mutually exclusive. From the foregoing information it can be seen that there is an interacting effect of essentially all of these factors involving the action of digitalis. The exact mechanism has not, as yet, been finally determined. Studies of the subcellular localization of administered digitoxin disclose that almost all of it is contained in the cytoplasmic portion of the cell, which contains the contractile protein as well as the transport system. .

Other Effects of Digitalis Administration

1. Digitalis therapy has no appreciable direct effect on coronary circulation. However, improvement of myocardial contractility may be reflected by changes in blood pressure and may also improve coronary circulation. Digitalis does cause some increase in the peripheral vascular resistance.

2. Digitalis has a mild direct diuretic action.

Metabolism

1. Cardiac glycosides are bound to plasma albumin to various degrees. The more rapid acting and rapidly excreted cardiac glycosides are bound to a lesser extent than the longer acting glycosides, as follows:
   a. Ouabain: not bound to plasma albumin.
   b. Cedilanid (lanatoside C): bound only to a slight degree.
   c. Digitoxin: bound to plasma albumin to an appreciable degree.

2. Plasma binding does not affect the ultimate action of cardiac glycosides on the heart.

3. Protein binding does not completely explain differences between the speed of action of the various cardiac glycosides.

4. The fate of cardiac glycosides in the blood stream is not completely known. Part of the digitalis is biotransformed.

5. Rates of elimination of digitalis glycosides vary widely.
   a. Excretion of both the unchanged glycosides and their degradation products occur chiefly through the kidneys.
   b. Presence of renal disease will alter the maintenance dose and in many instances the digitalizing dose. (Watch for azotemia and uremia.)

Indications and Contraindications for Digitalis

INDICATIONS

1. Congestive heart failure. If VPCs are a manifestation of congestive heart failure, digitalis may abolish them. VPCs may also be the manifestation of ventricular irritability via acute myocardial infarction or digitalis toxicity.

2. Pulmonary edema.

3. Atrial fibrillation. Direct action on AV conduction system to increase the refractory period, thereby slowing the rate of impulse conduction. (Slows ventricular rate.)

4. Atrial flutter. Action as in atrial fibrillation. Also,

digitalis increases the AV block which already exists in atrial flutter. (Slows ventricular rate.)

5. Paroxysmal supraventricular tachycardia. Action is by means of increased vagal tone and the effects on the SA node in the presence of the higher doses necessary to terminate this arrhythmia.

6. Cardiogenic shock. Many physicans now administer digitalis to patients in shock following acute myocardial infarction even in the absence of obvious congestive heart failure. The purpose is to receive the benefits of the inotropic action of digitalis.

7. To control arrhythmias secondary to heart failure.

CONTRAINDICATIONS

Contraindications to cardiac glycoside therapy are related to the toxic manifestations of digitalis and to the mechanism of action of digitalis on the electrical impulse apparatus of the heart. There are numerous *relative* contraindications to digitalis; however, there are few *absolute* contraindications. Some of the more stringent contraindications as well as factors to consider regarding continuation of therapy are given here.

1. Recent or current administration of digitalis.
   a. A careful history of digitalis ingestion, the specific agent and the last therapy by that agent is an important prerequisite to digitalis administration.
   b. An ECG should be taken before digitalization if possible, as occasionally unexpected digitalis toxicity may be revealed. This will usually already have been done in the acute coronary care situa-

tion. A current ECG prior to therapy is desirable.

2. Continuation of digitalis maintenance and adjustment of digitalis dose also depend on an exact history of previous digitalis therapy.
   a. Any arrhythmia due to cardiac glycoside therapy and not due primarily to acute myocardial infarction is a contraindication to digitalis therapy.
   b. This distinction may frequently be difficult to make, and the accurate history of previous digitalis therapy is again of extreme importance in distinguishing the cause of arrhythmias.

3. In the absence of previous digitalis therapy, ventricular tachycardia is the only *absolute* contraindication to digitalis administration, and in the face of cardiogenic shock this contraindication may not be absolute. The administration of cardiac glycosides in the presence of other arrhythmias in the patient suffering acute myocardial infarction is dependent on the specific arrhythmia and/or the manifestation of congestive heart failure, pulmonary edema or cardiogenic shock.
   a. Any arrhythmia in which the cardiac output is decreased may well benefit from digitalis therapy. Other medications being administered and the clinical circumstances must be taken into account.
   b. Even in the presence of AV block and associated decreased cardiac output and shock, digitalis therapy may be indicated. Other therapy, namely, electrode catheter pacing of the right ventricle and other medical therapy, is primarily indicated before digitalis.

Administration, Preparations and Dosage

PRINCIPLES OF ADMINISTRATION

Digitalis is given in an initial digitalizing dose, which is the amount needed to obtain therapeutic effects in a patient not previously receiving the drug; and in a maintenance dose, which is the amount needed for a given time interval to maintain these therapeutic effects.

As each patient has an individual digitalizing dose and maintenance dose, and as any given person may have varied organ system disease, the individual initial and maintenance doses of digitalis are quite variable. Therefore, the doses for each patient must be *titrated* in order to achieve the individual digitalizing and maintenance dosage.

The physician will benefit by being thoroughly familiar with the more commonly used preparations (e.g., Cedilanid, ouabain and Digoxin for intravenous use and Digoxin, digitoxin and gitalin for oral use). So long as the proper dosage is administered, one is not specifically more effective than the other in the hands of an individual physician. Intravenous administration has no advantage over oral administration except in an emergency situation when rapid action of the preparation is imperative.

ROUTES OF ADMINISTRATION

Cardiac glycosides may be administered by the oral route, intramuscularly or intravenously. The route of administration and the utilization of specific cardiac glycosides depend on the rapidity with which digitalization must be accomplished (the emergency nature of the situation). For details of preparations and routes of administration see Table 4.

1. If the IV route is used, ouabain, Cedilanid and digoxin are preferable.
2. With oral administration some digitalis preparations are not dependably absorbed from the gastrointestinal tract.
3. In general, IM administration is not considered thoroughly dependable with regard to rapidity and completeness of absorption.

Preparations Available for Clinical Use

Which preparations to use? Limit the number. It is impractical for any single physician to be adequately familiar with all the available preparations, routes of administration and doses for all cardiac glycosides.

TABLE 4.—Preparations and Routes of Administration of Digitalis

Digitalis Preparation	Oral	IM	IV	Comments
Powdered digitalis	X			
Digitalis tincture	X			
Ouabain (G-strophanthin)			X	
Digitoxin	X	X	X	
Digoxin	X	X	X	
Lanatoside C	X			
Deslanoside (desacetyl lanatoside C, Cedilanid-D)		X	X	Same pharmacologic properties as lanatoside C; available injectable form of lanatoside C
Digilanid	X			Available as rectal suppositories
Acetyldigitoxin	X			
Gitalin	X			
Digalen	X		X	
Digifolin	X		X	

Therefore, most physicians become familiar with a limited number of digitalis preparations.

1. Usually ouabain, Cedilanid or Digoxin is used for rapid IV digitalization in the acute coronary care unit. Numerous preparations are available for oral and IM utilization.
2. Factors to be considered in selecting a digitalis preparation are:
   a. Intestinal absorption.
   b. Speed of onset of action.
   c. Duration of cardiac action.
   d. Likelihood of emesis from local irritation.
   e. Stability and uniform potency of the preparation.
   f. Margin of safety.

DOSAGE SCHEDULES SUGGESTED FOR IV DIGITALIZATION

Initial digitalization in the acute coronary care unit is of necessity frequently accomplished by IV digitalization, using individual preparations as follows:

1. Digoxin (Lanoxin): 0.75 mg. initial IV dose; follow with 0.25 mg. IV every 1–4 hours until the patient is digitalized.
2. Deslanoside (Cedilanid-D): 0.8 mg. IV initially, followed by increments of 0.2–0.4 mg. every 1–4 hours to a total of 1.6 mg. or until the desired clinical effect is achieved.
3. Strophanthin (ouabain): 0.1 mg. IV approximately every 10–20 minutes to a total dose of 0.3–0.4 mg. IV in 90 minutes, or 0.7 mg. in 24 hours.

Table 5 presents in tabular form the rapid digitalization dosage of some of the commonly used digitalis preparations as well as their routes of administration, the time until effect, excretion and toxicity.

SPECIAL FACTORS MODIFYING DOSAGE

1. Previous therapy with cardiac glycosides. It is essential that a history for previous digitalis ingestion be obtained and that the type of cardiac glycoside preparation and the length of time since last administered be known and evaluated.
2. Acute myocardial infarction. There has been some evidence from animal experiments to indicate that the infarcted myocardium manifests an increased sensitivity to digitalis preparations. It is felt, therefore, that digitalis should be given only in reduced amounts. Many authorities administer approximately 75% of the usual average digitalizing dose to the patient with acute myocardial infarction when digitalis is being administered for the purposes of increasing myocardial contraction and cardiac output.[14,15,16]
3. Supraventricular tachycardia, auricular fibrillation and auricular flutter. In the presence of these arrhythmias, approximately 125% of the usual digitalizing dose is frequently required to convert the arrhythmia. Use of this dosage must be approached with caution, and if the arrhythmia is converted, toxic manifestations and secondary arrythmias due to the drug itself must be anticipated. Determination of whether the arrhythmia is due to acute myocardial injury or to the digitalis preparation may be difficult.
4. Elderly patients. Since kidney function is frequently decreased in the elderly, as manifested by a decrease in creatinine clearance, and since digitalis is excreted by the kidneys, the elderly patient may require a lower initial digitalization dose and a lower maintenance dose.
   a. In one study of Digoxin[167] it was found that higher blood concentrations and longer blood half-life occurred in the elderly. This was felt to be due to the generally smaller body size and the diminished urinary excretion of Digoxin in the elderly.

TABLE 5.—Rapid Digitalization; Comparative Chart of Digitalis Preparations

	DESLANOSIDE (Cedilanid-D)	STROPHANTHIN (Ouabain)	DIGOXIN	DIGITOXIN	GITALIN
Method of Administration					
Very Rapid, IM or IV (12 Hrs. or Less)	0.8 mg. stat; 0.4 mg. in 30–60 min. Follow by 0.4 mg. 2 hr. later. Add 0.2 mg. increments q 2 hr. as needed. IV and IM dose same	IV only. 0.3–0.5 mg. stat. Follow by 0.1–0.2 mg. q 30 min. to maximum dosage of 1 mg. in 24 hr. Other dosage schedules (text)	0.5–0.75 mg. stat. Follow by 0.25 mg. in 1–2 hr. Add 0.25 mg. increments q 1–2 hr. as indicated until effect or toxicity. IV and IM dose same	0.8 mg. initially, 0.2 mg. q 6–8 hr. until digitalized	2.5 mg. initially, then 0.75 mg. q 6 hr. until digitalized
Oral (12–24 Hr.)	Follow IV or IM with full digitalization dosage of a slower-acting preparation after acute digitalizing effect is obtained. Titrate	Follow with full digitalization dosage of slower-acting preparation.	1.5 mg. initially, then 0.5 mg. q 6 hr until digitalized		
Time of Action					
Onset of Effects	10–30 min. (IV route)	3–10 min. (IV route)	5–30 min. (IV route) Within 1 hr. (oral route)	2–4 hr.	2–4 hr.
Maximum Effects	1–2 hr.	1/2–2 hr.	1-1/2–5 hr.	12–24 hr.	8–10 hr.
Action Regressing	16–36 hr.	8–10 hr.	8–10 hr.	2–3 days	
Duration of Effects (Action Gone)	3–6 days	1–3 days	2–6 days	2–3 wks.	
Average Digitalizing Dose					
IV or IM (Less than 12 Hr.)	1.0–2.0 mg.	IV only: 0.6–1.0 mg.	0.75–1.0 mg.	1.0–2.0 mg.	5.0 mg.
Oral (12–24 Hr.)			2.0–4.0 mg.	1.0–2.0 mg.	0.25–1.0 mg.
Oral Maintenance Dose			0.25–1.0 mg.	0.5–2.0 mg.	
Duration of Toxicity	1–2 days, often gone within hours	2–6 hr.	1–2 days, often gone within hours	3–14 days	3–7 days
Elimination Rate	Rapid 2–3 days	Rapid 2–3 days	Rapid 3 days	Slow 2–3 weeks	Slow 7–10 days
Precautions and Comments	Monitoring preferred. Initial 0.8 mg. safe dose. Dosage may be varied following this dose. One of drugs of choice	Monitor ECG because effects are variable. Initial dosage schedules variable. One of drugs of choice	After IV or IM digitalization, continue with oral maintenance. One of drugs of choice. Felt by many to be equivalent of Cedilanid IM form causes severe local pain; may limit IM use.	Long period of elimination. Not recommended in acute myocardial infarct for rapid IV or IM initial digitalization due to slower onset of action and slower elimination	Slow elimination. Not recommended for acute infarction or for IV use. Dose variable

1) Serum creatinine tests did not permit prediction of this situation, since creatinine clearance can decrease more than 50% before there is a significant rise in serum creatinine concentration. Therefore, decreased Digoxin clearance was frequently found in the elderly with normal or near normal concentrations of serum creatinine.

2) Elevation of blood urea nitrogen (BUN) or nonprotein nitrogen (NPN) values represents evidence of renal damage in most instances. When one of these values is elevated, the digitalizing and maintenance doses of digitalis must be carefully titrated, and are usually lower.

5. Renal function. Chronic renal disease may alter the required digitalization and maintenance doses for cardiac glycosides since the major route of digitalis excretion is the kidneys and little of the drugs are inactivated by biotransformation. Renal function and glycoside kinetics are the basis for determining predictable daily maintenance doses of digoxin.[94] Use less digitalis in the presence of azotemia.

6. Decompensation. Clinically, lower resistance to digitalis toxicity is seen in a patient with cardiac decompensation who is taking diuretics, with the result that therapeutic dosage and toxic dosage are in the same general range.

7. Concurrent use of other drugs.
   a. Quinidine and procainamide (see Chapter 9). Combinations of these drugs with digitalis may increase the probability of digitalis toxicity.
   b. Diuretics. The concurrent use of diuretics and digitalis increases the probability of digitalis toxicity, the tolerance for digitalis being lower when diuretics are used. This effect is due to the lowering of potassium level caused by the diuretic action.
   c. Potassium. Low serum potassium content is associated with digitalis toxicity, and replacement of potassium is one of the mainstays in therapy of digitalis toxicity.
   d. Calcium. Myocardial actions of calcium and digitalis are similar and calcium may precipitate arrhythmias, including ventricular fibrillation, in digitalized patients. Intravenous administration of calcium should be avoided with digitalis therapy. (Obviously in cardiopulmonary resuscitation this need not apply as myocardial irritability is the desired goal of calcium injection in this situation.)
   e. Magnesium. Magnesium sulfate has been tried in treatment of digitalis intoxication. However, the effects are too transient to be useful clinically. Magnesium salts depress the contractility of cardiac as well as skeletal muscle but have little effect on the normal electrocardiograph.

f. Ephedrine and epinephrine. These drugs and digitalis may prove more toxic when given together than when the same dose of either is used alone.
   g. Isoproterenol (Isuprel). Digitalis and isoproterenol in combination increase the likelihood of digitalis toxicity and myocardial irritability.
   h. Other sympathomimetics. These agents in general cause increased likelihood of toxicity when used with digitalis therapy.

Digitalis Effects on ECG: Clinical Significance

Electrocardiographic changes cannot in themselves be regarded as an index of the degree of digitalization; however, they may serve to confirm clinical impressions of digitalis intoxication. Certain changes are usually associated with the therapeutic effects of cardiac glycoside therapy and certain ECG changes are most usually associated with toxic effects of digitalis therapy.

THERAPEUTIC EFFECTS

Below are some of the ECG changes that may represent the effects of digitalis rather than the effects of acute myocardial infarction, though the differentiation is frequently difficult. Continue cardiac glycoside therapy as indicated by the clinical condition under these circumstances.
1. Sagging ST segment.
2. Lowered T-wave (seen in acute myocardial infarction).
3. Shortened QT interval.
4. Prolonged PR interval during sinus rhythm (0.2–0.3 seconds).
5. Slowing of ventricular rate with rapid atrial arrhythmias even with occasional nodal escape.
6. Change from atrial tachycardia to atrial fibrillation or flutter.

TOXIC EFFECTS

Cardiac glycosides should be temporarily discontinued *if the following develop:*
1. Regularization of atrial fibrillation.
2. Acceleration of sinus tachycardia.
3. Paroxysmal atrial tachycardia, with latent or evident AV block.
4. Intermittent or sustained AV dissociation.
5. Second degree or complete AV block.
6. SA block with nodal rhythm, retrograde conduction and reciprocal beats.
7. Nodal tachycardia.
8. Ventricular premature complexes.
9. Bigeminal rhythm.
10. Ventricular tachycardia.

Digitalis Intoxication

GENERAL CONSIDERATIONS

All digitalis preparations cause signs and symptoms of intoxication when given in high enough doses. There are no "nontoxic" cardiac glycosides. The toxic manifestations of glycosides that are more rapidly excreted will be more rapidly dissipated, but the danger of toxicity is present with all preparations. The effects of digitalis toxicity on the heart can be lethal. It is the obligation of each physician who uses any preparation of the cardiac glycosides to be alert to those signs and symptoms of toxicity that call for cessation of therapy. In animals the lethal dose is probably in the range of 5–10 times the minimally effective therapeutic dose. In man the lethal dose is in the range of *only* about twice the dose which causes minor toxic manifestations. Therefore, the drug given in amounts adequate to cause maximum therapeutic effects has a *narrow remaining margin of safety.*

Digitalis intoxication presents a potentially life-threatening situation to a patient with acute myocardial infarction. The problem of whether or not the symptoms are due to digitalis intoxication, to the disease process or to other medications is nearly always present. Arrhythmias which occur with digitalis intoxication also occur with acute myocardial infarction, and some of these arrhythmias are treated with digitalis. Suggested steps to follow in determining and treating digitalis intoxication are:

1. If digitalis has not been administered during the hospital stay and digitalis intoxication is suspected, re-evaluate information from the patient and/or relatives concerning digitalis or "heart medicines," diuretics or "fluid pills" and previous medical contact within the past month.
2. Obtain a standard ECG.
3. Determine the serum electrolytes, in particular serum potassium and BUN or NPN.

TOXIC MANIFESTATIONS OF CARDIAC GLYCOSIDES[7,10,38,72,77]

The following listing of the toxic manifestations of cardiac glycosides represents the effects on various organ systems. However, the system in which the toxic manifestations of digitalis occur is not necessarily the organ system in which these manifestations are initiated. For example, anorexia is a gastrointestinal symptom having a central nervous system origin in the emetic center.

The gastrointestinal symptoms and the cardiac effects of cardiac glycoside toxicity are relatively closely correlated. The noncardiac side effects of digitalis toxicity are important because they may precede cardiac effects.

Gastrointestinal Effects

1. Anorexia is usually the earliest gastrointestinal manifestation.
   a. Anorexia is caused by central nervous system reflex action on the vomiting mechanism.
2. Nausea and vomiting.
   a. Do not rely on anorexia, nausea or vomiting alone as symptoms of overdigitalization.
3. Diarrhea.
4. Abdominal discomfort or pain.

Neurologic Effects

1. Mental depression in an otherwise cheerful patient is frequently one of the first manifestations seen.[38]
2. In elderly patients peripheral neuritis can be an early sign.
3. Manifestations of cerebral excitation.
   a. Headaches.
   b. Vertigo.
   c. Increased irritability and restlessness.
   d. Dizziness.
4. Drowsiness.
5. Confusion and fatigue.
6. Abnormal visual changes.
   a. Changes in color vision (especially yellow and green, white vision, frosted vision, halo effect).
   b. Restricted visual fields accompanied by a band-like headache.[38]
   c. Scotomas.
   d. Blurred or dim vision.
   e. Flickering lights, flashing of light, photophobia.
   f. Transient amblyopia, diplopia (paresis of ocular muscles), optic neuritis, oscillatory movements of eyeballs—absolute contraindication to further administration.
7. Less common neurologic manifestations: paresthesias, euphoria and amnesia, stupor, convulsions, coma.

Cardiovascular Effects

1. Ventricular premature contractions is usually the first arrhythmia to appear.[38]
2. Ventricular tachycardia.
3. Increased heart rate may be first evidence of digitalis toxicity.[7,77]
4. Atrial tachycardia—with or without AV block.
5. Nodal tachycardia—with or without AV dissociation.
6. AV blocks or any AV conduction disturbance.
7. Atrial fibrillation.
   a. Beware of regular ventricular rhythms—fast or slow—in the presence of auricular fibrillation (i.e., complete AV block with nodal rhythm).
   b. Observe for potassium deficiency due to combinations of digitalis and diuretics if auricular fibrillation occurs via digitalis toxicity.

8. Digitalis toxicity is considered to occur if digitalis is being administered in the presence of auricular fibrillation and there is:
   a. No slowing of ventricular rate after digitalis administration.
   b. An increase in ventricular rate—regular or irregular.
   c. A decided slowing of ventricular rates with:
      1) Occurrence of sinus rhythm (conversion).
      2) Continued auricular fibrillation.
9. Sinus arrhythmia, sinus arrest, SA block, atrial standstill.
   a. Via vagal action causing decreased SA impulse formation or conduction.
10. Nodal rhythm, nodal tachycardia or interference beats.

Other Effects

1. Allergic manifestations, such as skin rash.
2. Gynecomastia, usually after longer term digitalis administration.

THERAPY OF DIGITALIS INTOXICATION

Digitalis intoxication may be treated by a variety of therapeutic measures. It may be beneficial to use a combination of medical therapies. If an arrhythmia has resulted from digitalis toxicity, combinations of medical therapy and electroconversion may be necessary. The toxicity may also depend on the presence of any of the special factors modifying digitalis effect.

If digitalis toxicity is suspected, the first measure is to discontinue digitalis administration until a definite decision is made concerning the presence or absence of digitalis toxicity.

Specific Measures

One or more of the following measures may be utilized, depending on the clinical manifestations.

Potassium Therapy. Hypokalemia, and the metabolic alkalosis which is often associated with it, increases susceptibility to digitalis toxicity. Because cardiac glycosides decrease the potassium content of the heart, digitalis intoxication is apt to occur in patients receiving therapeutic doses of cardiac glycosides and diuretics simultaneously. Thus, if both digitalis and diuretics were used before the acute myocardial infarction, it may well be necessary to administer potassium, particularly if the serum potassium level is found to be low. In this circumstance the following potassium therapy should be carried out:

1. Administer 40 mEq. potassium chloride in 500 ml. of 5% D/W.
   a. Give at a constant rate of infusion, so as not to introduce erratic amounts into the circulation.
   b. Give over a period of not less than 1 hour.
2. Potassium therapy should not be used in the face of AV block.
3. If metabolic alkalosis is present and the levels of serum chlorides are lowered, the chloride salt of potassium must be used (oral or IV); otherwise it is difficult to correct the potassium deficit.

Diphenylhydantoin (Dilantin). Give 100 mg. slowly IV at the rate of 10 mg./minute, titrated.

Propranolol (Inderal). Propranolol can be given by various routes:

1. Intravenous: 1–3 mg. IV, slowly (for digitalis-induced tachycardia).
2. Oral: 20 mg. orally 4 times daily, increasing to 120–200 mg. daily.
3. Contraindicated in the presence of bronchial asthma, congestive heart failure, AV or bundle branch block[15] (except supraventricular tachycardia with block).

Lidocaine (Xylocaine). In the presence of appropriately treatable arrhythmias:

1. Give lidocaine 1–2 mg./kg. IV bolus followed by 1–2 mg./minute IV.
2. Use in ventricular arrhythmias, particularly refractory ventricular tachycardia, and before cardioversion[15] of any digitalis-induced arrhythmia.

Procainamide or Quinidine. Avoid in AV block. In patients with digitalis intoxication, quinidine may cause ventricular tachycardia, ventricular fibrillation and sudden death. If AV block is present quinidine may induce ventricular standstill.

Cardioversion of Digitalis-Induced Arrhythmias. Cardioversion as the sole means of therapy of digitalis-induced ventricular arrhythmias has been both fairly unsuccessful and likely to cause more serious arrhythmias or cardiac arrest.[263,264] Animal experiments utilizing countershock alone in the presence of digitalis intoxication[19,39,263] have indicated that countershock almost invariably failed to terminate or even interrupt the ventricular arrhythmias and frequently caused further myocardial irritability. However, the use of synchronized DC countershock in ventricular tachycardia *pretreated with lidocaine* resulted in a much less frequent occurrence of additional hazardous arrhythmias. Cardioversion under these circumstances was successful in a number of instances, that is, after lidocaine pretreatment. Lidocaine administered alone without countershock may be preferable to lidocaine followed by countershock therapy.

CHAPTER 13

Diuretics

The primary hemostatic role of the kidneys is to maintain the balance of water, electrolytes and other solutes in the body. The mechanism of this hemostatic regulation is by urinary excretion and conservation of the appropriate materials. Diuretics are drugs which increase urine volume.

The subject of renal physiology will not be dealt with here. Excellent presentations of the subject, adequate for the understanding of diuretic action, are available.[7,14]

PATHOLOGIC PHYSIOLOGY

When the onset and development of heart failure are slow enough for the process to be called congestive heart failure, the kidney tubule reabsorbs excessive amounts of electrolyte and increased extracellular fluid accumulates (edema, pulmonary engorgement). Three therapeutic approaches are available to mobilize the fluid and maintain extracellular fluid volume.

1. Restore competency of myocardial contraction.
2. Assist the kidney in suppressing tubular reabsorption by the use of drugs (the diuretics).
3. Reduce the amount of sodium salts absorbed from the gastrointestinal tract.
   a. This is accomplished by reducing the sodium intake.

MECHANISM OF ACTION; CLASSIFICATION OF DIURETICS

The diuretic agents include a number of drugs. These agents may be classified into 3 groups according to the mechanism of action. These groups, as well as their general subgroups, are as follows:[7,14]

1. Agents which increase renal plasma flow and glomerular filtration rate.
   a. Theophylline and aminophylline (theophylline ethylenediamine).
2. Agents which increase solute excretion of glomerular filtrate and tubular fluid.
   a. Osmotic diuretics.
      1) Mannitol.
      1) Urea.
3. Agents which inhibit renal tubular transport and sodium reabsorption.
   a. Organic mercurials.
   b. Benzothiadiazides (thiazides) and related sulfamyl diuretics.
   c. Carbonic anhydrase inhibitor (acetazolamide sodium, Diamox).
   d. Aldosterone inhibitor (spironolactone, Aldactone).
   e. Miscellaneous group.
      1) Triamterene (Dyrenium).
      2) Ethacrynic acid (Edecrin).
      3) Furosemide (Lasix).

The generic and trade names of the commercially available diuretics are available in several sources.[7,10,14] Literature concerning the pharmacology of these various drugs is also available.[7,10]

Diuretic Therapy in Acute Coronary Care

INDICATIONS

1. Many patients are taking diuretic agents to control congestive heart failure prior to acute myocardial infarction; therefore, their use and effect before and after myocardial injury must be evaluated.
2. In a patient with congestive heart failure following acute myocardial infarction diuretics are frequently a part of the total therapy.
3. Pulmonary edema necessitates the use of diuretic agents, usually of the more potent IM or IV agents (aminophylline, organic mercurials, furosemide and ethacrynic acid).

CONTRAINDICATIONS

1. Known hypersensitivity to the specific diuretic being considered.

102

a. This does not prevent substitution of a diuretic drug from another group.
2. Renal shutdown.
3. Azotemia—a relative contraindication. In congestive heart failure, diuretics may improve renal function and urine output. Check electrolytes frequently in this situation.
4. In the emergency situations requiring use of diuretics in acute coronary care there are few contraindications.

DIURETICS AND DIGITALIS TOXICITY

1. See Digitalis Intoxication in Chapter 12.
2. Digitalis causes a decrease in serum potassium, and diuretics also lower serum potassium levels.
3. In combination, digitalis and diuretics will frequently cause digitalis toxicity via decreased serum potassium.
4. When serum potassium is decreasing, the chloride ion is concomitantly carried out of the kidneys with the potassium ion. This loss creates a metabolic alkalosis. If chloride is not replaced along with potassium in patients with metabolic alkalosis, the potassium replacement will not be effective.
5. Therefore, if low serum potassium and chloride levels are found, the *chloride salt* of potassium *must* be administered, since hypokalemia will not be corrected by oral administration of other salts of potassium in this circumstance.
   a. Metabolic alkalosis is particularly apt to occur with the newer, more potent IV diuretics.

Specific Diuretics

It would not be realistic in this limited space to attempt to discuss all the individual diuretics. A few of the diuretic classes in general and the specific agents classified in the miscellaneous group will be discussed here as they may have been utilized before admission to the coronary care unit or during therapy of the patient in the acute coronary care unit. The following will be discussed.

1. Organic Mercurials.
2. Thiazides and related sulfamyl compounds.
3. Triamterene (Dyrenium).
4. Ethacrynic acid (Edecrin).
5. Furosemide (Lasix).

Organic Mercurials

Drugs of this group include, among others, meralluride (Mercuhydrin) and mercaptomerin sodium (Thiomerin sodium). The pharmacology of all are so similar they can be discussed as a group.

MECHANISM OF ACTION

Primary action decreases reabsorption of sodium and fixed anion by tubules.

DRUG EXCRETION

Largely and rapidly excreted by the kidney, thus avoiding mercurial toxicity. Caution in chronic kidney disease with azotemia.

ADMINISTRATION

Intramuscular route is the most desirable; oral administration is probably undesirable. No subcutaneous or IV administration.

CONTRAINDICATIONS

Renal insufficiency, because of possible systemic mercury poisoning and renal lesions which can be caused by these agents in this situation.

TOXIC REACTIONS

Numerous toxic reactions are possible but seldom occur. These include:
1. Rare, immediate fatal reactions after accidental IV administration.
2. Numerous gastrointestinal and skin reactions.
3. Systemic mercury poisoning with long-term use of oral preparations.
4. Depletion of extracellular electrolytes (not limited to mercurial diuretics).

Thiazides (Benzothiadiazides) and Related Sulfamyl Compounds[7,10,14]

DESCRIPTION

The thiazide diuretics are the most popular drugs for the long-term therapy of the edematous patient.

All thiazides examined to date have a similar mechanism of action. The various analogs differ primarily in the dose required to produce a given effect. There is a large number of thiazide analogs on the market (Diuril, Hydrodiuril, etc.).

MECHANISM OF ACTION

These compounds have a direct action on the renal tubular transport of sodium and chloride, and they may or may not have carbonic anhydrase inhibition, depending on the particular analog.

The dominant action is to increase the renal excretion of sodium and chloride and an accompanying volume of water. The renal effect is essentially independent of alterations in acid-base balance. The thiazides also cause a significant increase in excretion of potassium in amounts sufficient to cause predictable hypokalemia.

The thiazides have a hypotensive action with long-term use.

DRUG EXCRETION

The thiazides probably undergo secretion in the proximal tubule of the kidney nephron. Most thiazide compounds are excreted within 3–6 hours.

ADMINISTRATION

The thiazides are absorbed from the gastrointestinal tract and owe their usefulness in long-term therapy mainly to their effectiveness by the oral route. They show an effect within 1 hour after oral administration.

DOSAGE

The thiazides are available as tablets for oral administration. The wide range of dosage is dependent upon the thiazide analog selected.

Thiazides are evenly distributed throughout extracellular fluid and concentrated only in the kidneys.

INDICATIONS

See *Description.*

CONTRAINDICATIONS

1. Hypokalemia—or concurrently correct the potassium deficit.
2. Renal impairment—administer with care.

THE RELATED SULFAMYL DIURETICS

Though not strictly speaking thiazides, these agents have a similar activity and therefore may be considered as part of the same group.

CLINICAL TOXICITY

Clinical toxicity is relatively rare and results from hypersensitivity or from the combination of thiazide pharmacologic activity and the underlying disease process.
1. Hypersensitivity reactions reported.
   a. Purpura, dermatitis with photosensitivity, depression of blood-forming elements.
   b. Mild hyperglycemia with prolonged drug therapy in latent diabetics.
   c. Pancreatitis, rarely observed.
   d. Borderline renal and/or hepatic insufficiency may

be unpredictably aggravated by thiazides. The mechanism is not understood.
   e. Cholestatic hepatitis.
   f. Elevation of uric acid levels, particularly in latent gout, due to decreased renal uric acid clearance.
   g. Elevation of serum calcium, simulating hyperparathyroidism. It is thought that patients with this manifestation may have latent hyperparathyroidism.
2. Pharmacologic activity.
   a. In most patients depletion of intracellular potassium does not develop to a significant degree.
   b. Lowering of plasma potassium level may provoke digitalis toxicity and hypokalemic skeletal muscle paralysis.
3. Effect on laboratory values. It can be seen from the foregoing that the use of thiazide diuretics may affect the blood levels of potassium, glucose, uric acid, calcium and possibly other values.

Triamterene (Dyrenium)

MECHANISM OF ACTION

Triamterene increases the excretion of sodium and chloride in approximately equal amounts. It does not augment potassium excretion and may decrease it. The drug inhibits the reabsorption of sodium and chloride. Triamterene may have its greatest usefulness in conjunction with other diuretic agents.

ADMINISTRATION

Administered by the oral route only.

ADVERSE EFFECTS

1. Hyperkalemia may occur.
2. BUN level may be increased.
3. Repeated BUN and potassium determinations are therefore necessary.
4. Blood dyscrasias have been reported.

Ethacrynic Acid (Edecrin)

Ethacrynic acid is a newer and extremely potent diuretic. The drug produces a marked and prompt diuresis in individually adequate dosage; it should therefore be used judiciously and only in selected patients. The prompt and predictable effectiveness of the agent by the IV route has made it an ideal adjunct in the therapy of acute pulmonary edema.[18]

MECHANISM OF ACTION

1. The compound appears to react with sulfhydryl groups in both the proximal and distal renal tubules. Its major action is exerted in the proximal nephron, probably in the ascending limb of Henle's loop.

2. Both sodium and chloride excretion are substantial, and chloride excretion exceeds that of sodium.
3. Urinary output is usually dose dependent, and in some patients there is a *very small* difference between the dose causing *no* diuretic effect and that which causes *maximal* diuresis. Dosage determination may therefore be difficult.
4. Sodium to potassium ratio of elimination is more favorable than with thiazides, but the profound diuresis may cause excess amounts of potassium to be excreted.

Drug Excretion

1. The drug does not accumulate in organs other than the liver, and its high concentration at that site may be attributed to its excretion in the bile.
2. It is also excreted by the kidney and undergoes proximal tubular secretion.
   a. A cysteine-conjugated metabolite has been found in the urine.

Indications

1. Congestive heart failure of intractable nature and/or fairly rapid development.
2. Pulmonary edema.
3. The other medical indications are edema due to renal disease, cirrhosis with ascites and other causes. The drug is much more potent than the mercurials or thiazides.

Contraindications

1. This drug is so potent that great care must be exercised in its use. The profuse diuresis caused by the agent in appropriate dosage, along with changes in renal clearance of certain solutes with concomitant electrolyte alterations, make it a potentially dangerous drug. Additional information concerning the drug may be found in other sources.[7,10,14,18]
2. Contraindicated in anuria. If increasing azotemia and/or oliguria occur during treatment, the drug must be discontinued.
3. Severe, watery diarrhea occurs in a few patients. If this occurs, the drug must be permanently discontinued.
4. Frequent serum electrolyte, BUN and uric acid determinations should be performed if therapy is prolonged. Electrolyte determinations should be done when the diuresis is profound, even if therapy is brief.
   a. Because of the loss of chloride and hydrogen ion, a hypochloremic alkalosis may occur. Potassium may also be depleted, and this situation is an indication for potassium chloride therapy.

Administration and Dosage

1. The drug may be given orally or IV.
2. After oral administration, the diuretic response reaches a peak in 1–2 hours and persists for 4–5 hours.
3. Oral doses ranging from 50 to 400 mg. daily may be given; maximal response occurs with a dose of about 200 mg./day.
   a. The drug is not cumulative, so it may be used every 6–8 hours without risk of carry-over effects.
   b. If there is time, it is advisable to initiate therapy with small doses and progress to the dosage that produces maximal diuresis. In pulmonary edema this may not be possible, and maximal response must be attempted with the initial dose.
4. Intravenously ethacrynic acid is given in doses of 25–50 mg. A peak effect occurs in 30–60 minutes and diuresis persists for several hours.
   a. If necessary, the IV dose may be repeated in 4–6 hours.
5. In 5–10 minutes after IV administration an increase in urinary volume is noted.

Toxicity

1. With profuse diuresis of the type necessary when treating patients in the acute coronary care unit, the major side effects which might be anticipated are:
   a. Weakness, muscle cramps, paresthesias, thirst, anorexia and signs of hyponatremia, hypokalemia and/or hypochloremic alkalosis. Rarely tetany has been reported.
      1) These may be accentuated by rigid salt restriction.
      2) During therapy with ethacrynic acid and furosemide, liberalization of salt intake and use of supplementary potassium chloride are often necessary.
   b. The renal clearance of uric acid is depressed as in thiazide therapy, and transient reversible hyperuricemia may be seen.
   c. Transient azotemia in patients with underlying renal disease occurs.
   d. Gastric intolerance and profuse watery diarrhea occur in some patients after oral doses.
      1) If diarrhea occurs, discontinue drug and do not readminister.
   e. In studies of ethacrynic acid compared with hydrochlorothiazide at similar dose levels of 200 mg. daily, responses of similar magnitude were observed for each. There were increases in pulse rate and in serum concentrations of urea nitrogen and uric acid, and there were decreases in body weight, recumbent and standing blood pressure and serum concentrations of potassium and chloride.[40]
   f. Ototoxic effects have occurred, with vertigo, deafness and tinnitus and a sense of fullness in the

ears following rapid diuresis. These effects have all been reversible in 1-24 hours.

g. Local irritation and pain and a rare instance of thrombophlebitis have been reported at the site of IV injection.

2. With long-term administration (and in some cases of short-term administration) the following toxic effects might be seen:

a. Gastrointestinal symptoms have appeared after 1-3 months of continuous therapy. These have included anorexia, malaise, abdominal discomfort or pain, dysphagia, nausea, vomiting and diarrhea.

b. Numerous other side effects, such as agranulocytosis and abnormal liver function tests, have been reported in seriously ill patients taking numerous other medications.

c. Skin rash, headache, fever, chills, blurred vision, fatigue, apprehension and confusion have occurred infrequently.

Furosemide (Lasix)

Furosemide is a sulfonamide derivative, related to but more potent than the thiazide diuretics. Its pharmacologic effects are similar to those of ethacrynic acid.

Furosemide acts at the same site as ethacrynic acid; milligram for milligram, it is half as potent as ethacrynic acid. Furosemide is thought less likely to cause massive and uncontrolled diuresis.[18] Given IM, furosemide has been found as effective as organic mercurials and without the rare toxic reactions of mercurials.[41]

MECHANISM OF ACTION

The same as that of ethacrynic acid.

DOSAGE AND ADMINISTRATION

1. Furosemide is given orally in doses of 40-1,800 mg./day. The effects are not cumulative, therefore one may use the dose which produces the best diuretic response.

2. An IM dose of 20-40 mg. may be given.

3. An IV dose of 10-20 mg. may be given slowly, or as a constant infusion, supplying 0.5-1.0 mg./minute (with a maximum of 20-40 mg.).

TOXICITY

See Toxicity under Ethacrynic Acid. Furosemide toxicity is roughly the same.

CHAPTER 14

Drugs Affecting the Central Nervous System

Hypnotics, Sedatives and Tranquilizers

A discussion of the effects of pain and anxiety has been briefly presented in Chapter 8, General Therapeutic Measures. Hypnotics, sedatives and tranquilizers are the agents used to decrease anxiety in patients with acute myocardial infarction. Included are drugs which produce relaxation and sleep. Mention has been made of the fact that narcotics and non-narcotic analgesic agents are used to control the pain, anxiety and apprehension associated with acute myocardial infarction.

It would be impractical to attempt to cover, with any degree of completeness, the broad subject of sedatives, hypnotics and tranquilizers in this manual. Therefore, brief mention will be made of the various groups of agents, of some individual agents and of the possible adverse reactions that may occur when these agents are administered in acute myocardial infarction or are given in association with other drugs utilized in acute myocardial infarction.

Drugs found beneficial in the treatment of psychiatric disorders also are frequently used to decrease anxiety in the patient suffering acute myocardial infarction.

DEFINITIONS

1. **Hypnotics and sedatives.** These drugs are basically soporific drugs. They tend to produce sleep. The modern sedative-hypnotic agents are actually general depressants, causing depression of a wide range of cellular functions in many vital organ systems.
2. **Tranquilizers.** This definition is necessarily artificial. Drugs that are tranquilizers are usually divided into "major" and "minor" tranquilizers, depending on whether they are used in treating psychoses or anxiety, respectively.

Hypnotics and Sedatives: Barbiturates

The barbiturates are general depressants, affecting several different organ systems. They are quite unspecific in their effects and are capable of depressing, in a reversible manner, a wide range of biologic functions.

The barbiturates are derivatives of barbituric acid. They are divided into long-acting, short- to intermediate-acting, and ultrashort-acting derivatives. The long-acting derivatives are essentially entirely excreted by the kidneys, the short- or intermediate-acting derivatives are detoxified by the liver and excreted by the kidney and the ultrashort-acting derivatives are essentially totally detoxified by the liver. A complete presentation of the pharmacology is available in other sources.[7]

Specific Actions

1. Induce sleep.
2. No analgesic action.
3. Potent respiratory depressants, affecting both respiratory drive and the central nervous system center responsible for the rhythmic character of respiratory movements.
4. No significant effect on cardiovascular system in hypnotic doses, except for a slight decrease in blood pressure and heart rate such as occurs in *normal sleep*.
5. Produce a sleep similar to natural sleep.
6. "Dependence" may develop with long-term use.

Preparations

There is a great array of barbiturate derivatives and trade names. The structural formulas for 21 such derivatives are shown in one reference source.[7] The choice of agent depends mainly on the duration of action desired. The dosage depends on the depth of sedative or hypnotic effect desired.

Interactions with Other Drugs

When barbiturates (specifically phenobarbital) are given along with other drugs in the treatment of acute myocardial infarction, the following effects must be anticipated:

1. Analgesics—may inhibit the effect of the analgesic.
2. Anticoagulant—may inhibit the action of the anticoagulant.
3. Antihistamine—drugs may inhibit each other.
4. Anti-inflammatory agent—may inhibit the anti-inflammatory agent.
5. Diphenylhydantoin (Dilantin)—may inhibit effects of diphenylhydantoin.
6. Hypnotic—may inhibit action of other hypnotic.
7. Narcotic analgesic—may potentiate respiratory depression.
8. Monamine oxidase inhibitor—may potentiate action of barbiturate.
9. Minor tranquilizer—additive effect with barbiturates.
10. Phenothiazine derivative, e.g., chlorpromazine—additive effect particularly on respiratory depression and circulatory stability.

Other Hypnotics and Sedatives

Whereas, as a group, the barbiturates, are probably still the most useful and versatile sedative-hypnotic drugs, there are a large number of compounds of diverse chemical and pharmacologic properties that have the ability to produce a nonspecific, reversible depression of the central nervous system. A complete listing of these compounds may be found in other sources.[7] Some of the compounds and their side effects are described here.

CHLORAL HYDRATE

This agent is quite irritating to the skin and mucous membranes, and the local irritation of the gastrointestinal tract accounts for the principal side effects of gastric distress, nausea and vomiting.

1. Chloral hydrate and an anticoagulant together may enhance the effect of the anticoagulant.
2. Monamine oxidase inhibitors with chloral hydrate potentiate the effects of chloral hydrate.

ETHCHLORVYNOL (PLACIDYL)

This tertiary acethlenic alcohol has a short latency to onset and a short duration of action. Onset of depression after oral dosage appears in one-half hour, maximal depression occurs in 1–1½ hours and the drug is no longer detectable in the blood in 3 hours. The hypnotic dose is 500 mg. and the sedative dose is 100 or 200 mg. 2 or 3 times daily.

PIPERIDINEDIONE DERIVATIVES

Glutethimide (Doriden)

The structure closely resembles that of phenobarbital.

1. Toxic doses produce both cardiovascular and respiratory depression.
2. The drug exhibits pronounced anticholinergic activity.
3. Glutethimide is entirely metabolized in the body.
4. With therapeutic doses, toxic side effects are rare; they consist of gastric irritation, headache and, infrequently, skin rashes. Symptoms of acute intoxication are similar to those of barbiturate poisoning, namely, respiratory depression.
5. Glutethimide with anticoagulants inhibits the effect of the anticoagulants.
6. Dose is 500 mg., repeated once in not less than 4 hours.

Methyprylon (Noludar)

1. In doses of 300 mg. the hypnotic effect of methyprylon is virtually indistinguishable from that produced by 200 mg. secobarbital.
2. Side effects are mild and infrequent, consisting of nausea and vertigo.
3. The toxicity of methyprylon for the cardiovascular system seems to be at least as great as that of the barbiturates.
4. In adults the oral hypnotic dose is 200–400 mg. The sedative dose is 50–100 mg. 3 or 4 times daily.

METHAQUALONE

1. Similar to barbiturates in its hypnotic effects. Dose of 150 mg. is equivalent to 200 mg. cyclobarbital.
2. Possesses other actions.
3. Anesthetic concentrations produce hypotension owing to a direct action on the heart.
4. Side effects occur in about 5% of patients.
5. Hypnotic dose is 150–300 mg. Sedative dose is 75 mg. 3 or 4 times daily.

Phenothiazine and Related Compounds (Major Tranquilizers)

THE PHENOTHIAZINE DERIVATIVES

1. See specific agents in therapy of cardiogenic shock, Chapter 5.
2. See drugs affecting the sympathetic nervous system, Chapter 15.
3. Excellent references available.[7]
4. There are numerous phenothiazine derivatives available. Chlorpromazine has been discussed in the sources given in 2 and 3.

Actions and Side Effects

1. Chlorpromazine (derivative) has alpha adrenergic blockade effect. It may precipitate shock if impending shock is present.
2. Possible adverse reactions may occur when phenothiazines are combined with other drugs.

a. With antihistamines—additive effect.

b. With antihypertensive—potentiates antihypertensive effect.

c. With reserpine—potentiates reserpine effect.

d. With barbiturate—enhances sedation. May cause *respiratory depression*.

e. With monamine oxidase (MAO) inhibitor—inhibits effects of MAO inhibitor.

f. With meperidine or morphine—enhances sedation. May *potentiate respiratory depression*.

g. Minor tranquilizers (Librium, Valium, Serax, etc.) —additive effect.

h. Thiazide diuretic—may cause shock via several mechanisms.

i. Tricyclic antidepressant—additive effect.

PHENOTHIAZINE/ANTIHISTAMINE DERIVATIVES (PROMETHAZINE)

1. Most drugs of this class are histamine antagonists. Promethazine was originally introduced for the management of allergic conditions.

2. Promethazine (Phenergan) has a wide spectrum of clinical usefulness, including sedation, therapy of motion sickness and antihistaminic therapy.

3. In acute coronary care, the chief uses of promethazine are to potentiate the analgesic and sedative effects of the narcotic-analgesic drugs, permitting greater effect of the latter at lower doses.

Precautions, Side Effects and Contraindications

1. Promethazine potentiates the effects of central nervous system depressants, including:
   a. Barbiturates.
   b. Morphine.
   c. Meperidine.
   d. Pentazocine.
   e. "Major" and "minor" tranquilizers.
   f. Other central nervous system depressants of any type.

2. The chief concern in potentiation of central nervous system depressant agents is respiratory depression and hypotension.

Dosage

1. For sedation, dosage is 12.5–25 mg.

2. In conjunction with narcotic-analgesics, dosage is 25–50 mg. every 4–6 hours.

3. Promethazine may be given orally, IM or IV. When given IV, concentration should not exceed 25 mg./ml. and the rate of injection should not exceed 25 mg./minute.

Drugs for Anxiety (Minor Tranquilizers)

BENZODIAZEPINE COMPOUNDS

1. Three benzodiazepine compounds are currently being marketed. These are chlordiazepoxide (Librium), diazepam (Valium) and oxazepam (Serax).

2. These compounds are utilized mainly for the treatment of anxiety and for skeletal muscle relaxation.

3. These agents have mild sedative effects. They have not only central actions but peripheral effects on the cholinergic and adrenergic systems, although the evidence for the peripheral actions has not been fully established.

4. Chlordiazepoxide (Librium) and diazepam (Valium) have both been mentioned as mild sedatives for the relief of anxiety in the patient with acute myocardial infarction.[16]

5. Diazepam (Valium) is also used when it is necessary to produce loss of consciousness prior to defibrillation in the conscious patient. For this use it is given by the IV route.
   a. See Arrhythmias, Chapter 4.
   b. See Cardioversion in Chapter 10.

6. Chlordiazepoxide and diazepam are available for both oral and parenteral use.

7. Dosage of each of these agents must be individualized.

8. The advantage of one of these agents over another is not well defined.

9. Psychologic and physical dependence of the type seen with the barbiturates has been reported.

Adverse Reactions

1. Rarely, variable effects on blood coagulation have been reported in patients given a benzodiazepine compound and an oral anticoagulant.

2. With barbiturates—there is an additive effect.

3. With alcohol, phenothiazines and tricyclic antidepressants—there is an additive effect.

4. With MAO inhibitor—there is enhanced sedation.

5. Known hypersensitivity to any of these agents is a contraindication.

6. Numerous reactions and side effects of various types have been reported with each of these agents.[10]

MEPROBAMATE (MILTOWN, EQUANIL)

1. Meprobamate is among the most popular drugs for the treatment of anxiety.

2. The pharmacologic effects of meprobamate are similar to those of the barbiturates. It is difficult to differentiate between the 2 types of drugs in clinical usage. In the acute coronary care unit, used in therapeutic doses, effects of meprobamate could be likened to those of the barbiturates.

3. Meprobamate has both a sedative effect and a skeletal muscle relaxation effect.
4. In ordinary doses, it appears to be as safe as, or safer than, the barbiturates.
5. Various allergic and hematologic disorders have been reported.
6. A hypotensive effect of the drug is commonly seen, being more pronounced in elderly individuals.
7. Acute toxicity from ingestion of large amounts may result in loss of consciousness, hypotensive reactions and shock, respiratory depression and death.

HYDROXYZINE (VISTARIL, ATARAX)

1. Hydroxyzine is a rapid-acting ataraxic with a wide margin of safety. It induces a calming effect in anxious, tense adults. Hydroxyzine is not a central nervous system cortical depressant, but may suppress activity in key regions of the subcortical area of the central nervous system.
   a. Skeletal muscle relaxation, antispasmodic properties and antihistaminic effects have been demonstrated.
2. Indications: anxiety and tension.
3. Contraindications: Hydroxyzine may potentiate effects of narcotics, barbiturates and the "major" and "minor" tranquilizers.
4. Dosage is 25–100 mg. every 4–6 hours orally, IM or IV.
   a. Care must be taken not to give subcutaneously or intra-arterially.

Adverse Reactions

1. Drowsiness may occur; this may be desirable.
2. Adverse reactions are rare.
3. The drug should not be given subcutaneously, or inadvertently by the intra-arterial route. When given undiluted IV, a small amount of intravascular hemolysis occurs. When the drug is diluted and given over 4 hours (100 mg. in 4 hours), hemolysis is not noticeable.
4. It would seem apparent that the oral or IM routes are preferable.

Antidepressants

DIBENZAZEPINE COMPOUNDS (TRICYCLIC ANTIDEPRESSANTS)

1. The dibenzazepine derivatives are imipramine (Tofranil) and amitriptyline (Elavil).
2. An excellent review of the pharmacology of these agents is presented elsewhere.[7]
3. The chief pharmacology of these agents is as follows:
   a. Antidepressant effects.
   b. Cholinergic blocking properties (anticholinergic activity).
   c. Cardiovascular effects.

Toxicity and Precautions for Use in Acute Coronary Patients

1. Most frequent untoward effects are atropine-like actions; tolerance develops.
2. Various types of cardiovascular difficulties have occurred.
   a. Orthostatic hypotension—the patient develops a tolerance for this effect.
   b. Myocardial infarction precipitated by these drugs has been reported, the mechanism being undetermined.
   c. Congestive heart failure has occurred during the course of treatment and has been attributed to the drugs.
   d. Toxic doses of imipramine may produce cardiac arrhythmias and tachycardia.
   e. Imipramine can cause negative inotropic effects on the heart.
   f. Electrocardiographic changes following use of imipramine consist of inversion or flattening of the T-waves.
3. The transition from depression to hypomanic or manic excitement has occurred in certain patients. Treat wih phenothiazines.
4. Dibenzazepine derivatives must NOT be administered concurrently with or shortly after treatment with MAO inhibitors. At least a week should elapse between the 2 drugs. The toxic signs and symptoms of overlapping therapy resemble those of atropine toxicity.

Narcotics and Analgesics

Narcotics are agents which produce sleep as well as analgesia, and which are addicting.

In almost all patients suspected of having acute myocardial infarction, one of the narcotic drugs is used initially. This is done chiefly because in most patients the presenting symptom and the reason the patient seeks medical assistance is *pain*. A marked degree of anxiety also accompanies the onset of the pain associated with acute myocardial infarction. (See section on Pain and Anxiety in Chapter 8.) Although many narcotics are available and may be used, the 3 agents most often used are:

1. Morphine sulfate.
2. Meperidine hydrochloride (Demerol).
3. Pentazocine lactate (Talwin—a non-narcotic).

Other analgesic drugs might be used in acute coronary care, either for nonrelated pain or for pain of lesser degree that may be due to nonrelated medical problems. An example of this type analgesic is codeine or propoxyphene hydrochloride (Darvon). References to these and other narcotic and/or analgesic agents may be found in other sources.[7,10] The pharmacology of the 3 more commonly used narcotic analgesics will be presented here.

Morphine*

DESCRIPTION

Morphine is probably the most important derivative of the phenanthrene alkaloids of opium. The chemical structure is complex. There are 2 hydroxy groups on morphine, 1 phenolic, the other alcoholic. These hydroxy groups are of basic importance for the actions of morphine. By altering one or more of these hydroxy groups, codeine, heroin and hydromorphone (Dilaudid) are derived.

ACTIONS

The actions of morphine have been extensively studied for many years, and as early as 1941 there were over 10,000 references in the literature.

Central Nervous System Effects

The narcotic action of morphine manifests its effects by causing analgesia, drowsiness, changes in mood and mental clouding.

1. **Relief of pain.** Pain relief is the outstanding effect. The perception of pain itself is not always decreased, even in patients who obtain satisfactory pain relief. However, the patient's ability to tolerate pain may be markedly increased even when the capacity to perceive the sensation is relatively unaltered.
   a. Thus the feature of pain as suffering must be taken into account, considering both the original sensation of pain and the patient's reaction to that sensation.
2. **Hypothalamic CNS effects.** Morphine and most narcotics produce a release of antidiuretic hormone and thus cause a decrease in urinary output, the effect being mediated by the hypothalamus.
   ACTH and pituitary gonadotropic hormone release is inhibited.
3. **Pupil.** Morphine causes constriction of the pupil in man. The exact mechanism of this action is not known.
4. **Respiration.** Morphine is a primary and continuous respiratory depressant by virtue of a direct action on the brain stem respiratory centers. Respiratory depression is descernible with doses too small to produce sleep or disturb consciousness, and *increases progressively* as the dose increases. Therapeutic doses in man depress all phases of respiratory activity. A slower rate of breathing is a prominent symptom. Morphine and related narcotics may pro-

duce irregular and periodic breathing in man, even after therapeutic doses.
5. **Nausea and emesis.**
   a. The nausea and emetic effects of morphine and its derivatives are caused by direct stimulation of a center in the medulla (brain stem) of the CNS.
   b. The emetic action of morphine and its derivatives are counteracted by phenothiazine derivatives and by nalorphine (Nalline).
      Note: The phenothiazine derivative chlorpromazine (Thorazine) may cause hypotension by virtue of its alpha adrenergic blockade action.
   c. Besides stimulating the previously mentioned center in the brain stem, morphine depresses the vomiting center. Therefore, after therapeutic doses of morphine are given (even if vomiting results), subsequent doses are not likely to cause vomiting.
6. **Cough reflex.** Morphine and the opiates are the most effective agents available for suppressing the cough reflex.
7. **Dyspnea.** Certain forms of dyspnea may be markedly relieved by opiates (morphine). The dyspnea of acute left ventricular failure and pulmonary edema may respond dramatically to IV morphine. The mechanism is by way of increased capacitance in the peripheral vascular system.

Cardiovascular Effects

1. In the supine patient *without* acute myocardial infarction, therapeutic doses of morphine have little, if any, effect on blood pressure, heart rate or rhythm.[10]
2. However, studies in patients with acute myocardial infarction and observation of many patients not specifically studied have shown that bradycardia may occur.[62,112,156,173] It is thought that possibly the bradycardia is mediated by a primary action on the vagus nucleus in the medulla, and a result of reflex CNS activity.[62,173] This bradycardia is usually corrected by atropine.
3. There is peripheral vasodilatation following morphine injection, and this effect is via a direct effect on the smaller blood vessels.
   When morphine was administered to patients with acute myocardial infarction,[62] calculated peripheral resistance fell in many instances, sometimes causing transient hypotension and sometimes more prolonged hypotension. This type of hypotension was amenable to gravitational changes: for example, raising the legs of the patient could cause an increase in blood pressure. There is a gravitational stress effect in patients without acute myocardial infarction also. It is suggested that any patient who has received morphine, particularly if suspected of having acute myocardial infarction, be transported in a supine position and that the legs definitely not be in a dependent position.

---

*References: 7, 10, 62, 112, 137, 156.

a. Morphine and other narcotics should be used with caution in patients who have a decreased blood volume. The concurrent use of a narcotic analgesic agent and a phenothiazine derivative will not only potentiate respiratory depression produced by the narcotic but will also result in a greatly increased risk of hypotension.

METABOLISM

Morphine rapidly leaves the blood and is concentrated in parenchymatous tissues, such as the kidney, lung, liver and spleen. Though skeletal muscle contains lower levels, because of its mass it contains the major fraction of the drug in the body. Morphine does not accumulate in the tissues, and 24 hours after the last dose, tissue levels are quite low.

Morphine is excreted in the urine, with small amounts of free morphine and larger amounts of conjugated morphine being found; 90% is excreted in the first 24 hours. About 20% of the morphine is excreted in the bile, and some of this eventually appears in the feces.

INDICATIONS

The indications for morphine in acute myocardial infarction are pain and the anxiety associated with pain.

CONTRAINDICATIONS

Contraindications to the use of morphine in acute myocardial infarction are relative. The pharmacologic effects and side effects which should be considered in administering morphine to a patient have been considered under the actions of morphine. A review of the pertinent ones follows:
1. Respiratory depression is a primary effect.
   a. Use with great caution in patients with cor pulmonale, as deaths following ordinary therapeutic doses have been reported.[7]
   b. Concurrent use of morphine and a phenothiazine derivative may cause respiratory depression of great degree. It also may cause hypotension via vasodilatation.
   c. Nalorphine (Nalline) is the antagonist for morphine.[10] Dosage of 5–10 mg. given IV increases respiratory rate in 1 or 2 minutes.
      1) Nalorphine alone has analgesic effects, but because it has a significant percentage of unpleasant side effects, it is not used as a primary analgesic. Nalorphine given *alone* may depress respiration.
2. The first dose may produce vomiting, which is undesirable in the presence of acute myocardial infarction. Doses thereafter are not so apt to cause vomiting if administered within 3–4 hours.
3. Bradycardia may occur [62,112,156,173] via CNS action.

a. Treat with IV atropine. (See Atropine in Chapter 9.)
4. Hypotension via vasodilatation may occur.
   a. Elevate the legs to autotransfuse with venous blood from the lower extremities.
   b. Transport the patient who has received morphine in the supine position.
   c. Use care in administering morphine and phenothiazine derivatives together, especially chlorpromazine.

DOSAGE

Give 10–15 mg. IM every 3–4 hours depending on continuation of pain and occurrence of side effects.

TOXICITY

See both Actions and Contraindications in this section.

Meperidine (Demerol)

DESCRIPTION

After morphine, meperidine[7,10,14,16] is the drug which is probably the most widely used at present. Like most other narcotic analgesics, meperidine exerts its chief pharmacological actions on the central nervous system.

ACTIONS

Meperidine has many pharmacologic similarities to morphine, and it is presumed that its mechanism of action is the same.

Central Nervous System Effects

Therapeutic doses of meperidine produce analgesia, sedation, euphoria, respiratory depression and other CNS effects comparable to those of morphine.
1. **Relief of pain.** Therapeutic doses act primarily by altering the reaction to pain, whereby patients are more comfortable even though they may continue to perceive painful stimuli.
2. **Respiration.** In equivalent analgesic doses meperidine depresses respiration to the same degree as morphine.
   a. Like morphine, meperidine decreases the sensitivity of (1) the brain stem respiratory centers to CO_2 and (2) the CNS pontine centers involved in respiratory rhythmicity.
   b. With meperidine, tidal volume is decreased while respiratory rate may be relatively unaffected. The respiratory rate may also be depressed.
   c. Respiratory depression can be antagonized by administration of nalorphine (Nalline) or levallorphan (Lorfan).
3. **Pupil.** Pupil size and reflexes are not usually affected.

4. **Labyrinth.** Meperidine appears to increase the sensitivity of the labyrinthine apparatus in man. (Vertigo may occur.)
5. **Cough reflex.** Meperidine does not affect the cough reflex to as great an extent as morphine.
6. **Other CNS effects.** Meperidine differs from morphine in that toxic doses may cause CNS excitation.

Cardiovascular Effects

In patients not suffering from acute myocardial infarction, therapeutic doses of meperidine have no significant untoward effects on the cardiovascular system, particularly in recumbent patients.
1. There is no effect on myocardial contractility or the electrocardiogram.
2. If given IV, meperidine may cause hypotension, as does morphine. Apparently this also occurs via peripheral vasodilatation and histamine release.
3. IM administration does not affect heart rate.
4. IV administration frequently produces an increase in heart rate that is sometimes alarming. This is due to the atropine-like (anticholinergic) effect of the drug.
5. Meperidine was first investigated as an atropine-like drug and has some atropine-like effects.[7,14]

METABOLISM

1. After IV administration, plasma levels decline rapidly for the first 1 or 2 hours, and more slowly thereafter.
2. About 40% of meperidine is bound to nondiffusable constituents of the plasma.
3. About one-third of administered meperidine can be accounted for in the urine as N-demethylated derivatives. (These derivatives are important in causing drug combination toxic reactions.)

INDICATIONS

Pain and the anxiety accompanying pain are the indications in acute myocardial infarction.

CONTRAINDICATIONS

1. Severe reactions may occur when meperidine is administered to patients receiving monamine oxidase (MAO) inhibitors. These reactions are characterized by excitation, delirium and convulsions, or by severe respiratory depression and cyanosis without hypotension. The reactions may be related to the metabolic products of meperidine.
2. With concurrent administration of antidepressants of the imipramine type (Tofranil), meperidine-induced respiratory depression may be enhanced.
3. Concurrent administration of meperidine in therapeutic doses and phenothiazines may cause marked exaggeration of the respiratory depressant effect, both in degree and duration of the effect.

4. Some phenothiazines may antagonize the analgesic effects of meperidine.
5. Care must be taken with administration of meperidine in circumstances in which hypotension, tachycardia or respiratory depression may be particularly harmful.
   a. In particular, close attention must be given to the dosage in these situations.

DOSAGE AND ADMINISTRATION

1. **Routes of administration.** Meperidine may be given orally, subcutaneously, IM or IV. Effects of specific routes are as follows:
   a. Onset of analgesic effect is prompt (within 10 minutes) after subcutaneous or IM administration. Duration of action is approximately 2–4 hours, being somewhat shorter than that for morphine and necessitating a shorter interval between injections for the relief of continuing pain.
   b. Analgesic effects are detectable in about 15 minutes after oral administration in experimentally induced pain.
   c. IV doses cause very rapid effects.
2. **Dosage**
   a. Usually 100 mg. is given parenterally.
      1) IV potentiates possible toxic effects.
      2) Subcutaneous administration causes irritation.
      3) Oral dosage is slower in effect.
      4) Thus it is usually given IM.
   b. 75–100 mg. of meperidine given parenterally is equivalent to 10 mg. of morphine by the same route.

TOXICITY

1. Overdosage may result in profound respiratory depression, coma and death or may produce tremors and convulsions.
2. Untoward effects include dizziness, sweating, euphoria, dry mouth, nausea, vomiting, weakness, visual disturbances, palpitation, dysphoria, syncope and sedation.
3. Over-all incidence of individual side effects is quite similar to that observed with equivalent doses of morphine.
4. When used in patients bordering on cardiogenic shock, the drug may precipitate actual shock.[16]
5. Antagonists for respiratory depression are:
   a. Nalorphine (Nalline) IV in a dose of 5–10 mg.
   b. Levallorphan (Lorfan), 0.5–1.5 mg. IV.

Pentazocine (Talwin)

DESCRIPTION

Pentazocine[10,95,96,222] is a synthetic drug and member of the benzazocine series (benzomorphan series). Pentazocine is a newer agent, is non-narcotic, and is not subject to narcotic controls.

ACTION

Central Nervous System and Cardiovascular Effects

1. Pentazocine produces both sedation and analgesia. It has been found to be a highly effective non-narcotic analgesic.[95]
2. Pentazocine has been compared with morphine—and the following findings have emerged:
   a. At comparable analgesic dosages pentazocine causes less respiratory depression than does morphine.[96] However, some respiratory depression can occur.
   b. In a series of 200 patients treated in the coronary care unit, using 60 mg. doses IM, the analgesic potency of pentazocine was found to be as effective as that of morphine.[222]
   c. There is less likelihood of bradycardia or hypotension occurring with pentazocine than with morphine. In fact, with fairly large amounts of pentazocine a rise in blood pressure and pulse rate has been observed.[222]

Dependence Potential

1. Pentazocine is not classified as a narcotic on the basis of findings in direct addiction tests and is not subject to narcotic controls.
2. Pentazocine does not substitute for morphine in subjects who are physically dependent on morphine and does not prevent withdrawal symptoms.
3. It appears, however, that the long term use of the drug is subject to abuse, and abrupt discontinuance of pentazocine following excessive use of the parenteral form has resulted in symptoms such as abdominal cramps, elevated temperature, rhinorrhea, restlessness, anxiety and lacrimation. These have occurred primarily in patients with a history of narcotic drug abuse.
   a. In acute coronary care it seems unlikely that this problem would occur.

Caution

Pentazocine has been found to be a narcotic antagonist, and for this reason should not be given to patients who have been taking large doses of narcotics over a period of time, as withdrawal symptoms may occur.[95]

1. Intolerance or untoward reactions are seldom observed after administration of pentazocine to patients who have received single doses of narcotics or who have had limited exposure to narcotics.

METABOLISM

About 50% of radioactive pentazocine appears in the urine of patients in 12 hours; and 70% appears in the urine of monkeys in 24 hours.[237]

INDICATIONS

The indications for pentazocine in acute myocardial infarction are the same as for the narcotics: pain and the anxiety accompanying pain.

CONTRAINDICATIONS

1. Known sensitivity to the drug.
2. Increased intracranial pressure or any pathologic brain condition in which clouding of the sensorium is undesirable (as with the narcotics).

DOSAGE AND ADMINISTRATION

1. **Availability.** Pentazocine (Talwin) is supplied in ampules containing 30 mg., 45 mg. and 60 mg. and in multiple dose vials of 10 ml., each 1 ml. containing 30 mg. pentazocine. Tablets for oral administration are available, with 50 mg. pentazocine per tablet.
2. **Equivalent dose.** 30 mg. parenteral dose of pentazocine is approximately equal in analgesic activity to parenteral doses of 10 mg. morphine or 75–100 mg. meperidine. The duration of action of pentazocine may be less than that of morphine.
3. **Routes and onset of action.** Parenterally pentazocine (Talwin) may be given subcutaneously, IM or IV.
   a. Pain relief usually occurs in 15–20 minutes after IM or subcutaneous injection.
   b. Pain relief occurs within 2–3 minutes after IV administration.
4. **Duration of action.** Analgesia usually lasts 3 hours or longer after a single injection.
5. **Treatment of overdosage or respiratory depression**
   a. Narcotic antagonists such as nalorphine are not effective respiratory stimulants for respiratory depression due to pentazocine.
   b. Parenteral administration of methylphenidate (Ritalin) is used for respiratory depression caused by pentazocine (Talwin) overdose.
6. Pentazocine has been used in 60 mg. parenteral doses with good results in acute coronary care.[222]
7. Talwin should not be mixed in the same syringe with soluble barbiturates because precipitation will occur.

ADVERSE REACTIONS

1. Nausea, the most frequent adverse effect, occurs in about 5% of patients.
2. Vertigo, dizziness or lightheadedness, vomiting and euphoria occurred in less than 5% of more than 12,000 patients who received the drug parenterally.
3. Respiratory depression was reported in about 1% of the patients.
4. The following adverse effects occurred in well below 1.0%: constipation, circulatory depression, diaphoresis, urinary retention, alteration in mood (nervousness, apprehension, depression, floating feeling), hypertension, sting on injection, headache,

dry mouth, flushed skin, dermatitis including pruritus, dreams, paresthesia and dyspnea.

5. The following adverse reactions occurred in less than 0.1% of the patients: tachycardia, visual disturbances (blurred vision, nystagmus, diplopia), hallucinations, disorientation, weakness or faintness, muscle tremor, chills, allergic reactions including edema of the face, taste alteration, insomnia, diarrhea and cramps, and miosis.

6. It must be noted from the low incidence of adverse reactions that this non-narcotic analgesic sedative is probably the least likely of the 3 drugs considered

to cause adverse effects in the acutely ill patient with acute myocardial infarction.

COMMENT

Although this agent seems to be the safest of the 3 drugs, it must be remembered that the drug has not been available very long. It was once thought that meperidine was much safer than we now know it to be, and wider use may provide more information concerning the use, contraindications and side effects of pentazocine.

CHAPTER 15

Drugs Affecting the Autonomic Nervous System

The Parasympathetic Nervous System

PARASYMPATHOLYTIC AGENTS

ATROPINE: This drug is a parasympatholytic (*vagal blocking*) agent. Description and properties are presented in Chapter 9.

PARASYMPATHOMIMETIC AGENTS[7,72,231]

1. **General effect.** The effect of parasympathetic stimulation is to *increase* vagal tone. This is accomplished via accentuation of normal physiologic mechanisms and by drug therapy.
2. **Vagal stimulation.** A transient increase in vagal tone may result from carotid sinus massage or by performing the Valsalva maneuver. These are the classic methods for attempting to convert supraventricular tachyarrhythmias. If increased vagal tone is not produced by these methods, drugs may be administered. It is worthwhile to note that, after administration of a parasympathomimetic agent, carotid sinus massage or the Valsalva maneuver are more likely to cause increased vagal tone.

EDROPHONIUM (TENSILON)

1. Edrophonium is a cholinergic drug which exerts its action by inhibiting cholinesterase, thus enhancing the effect of endogenous acetylcholine. Its effect is that of vagal stimulation.
2. This agent has been widely utilized to obtain intense and transient vagal stimulation for the following purposes:
   a. Differentiating atrial tachyarrhythmias. If the ventricular rate responds to the drug, this strongly suggests that the arrhythmia is of supraventricular origin. Also, slowing of the ventricular rate sometimes permits previously obscured P-waves to become visible, thus permitting ECG diagnosis of the arrhythmia.
   b. Converting supraventricular tachyarrhythmias. The drug has had transient responses on supraventricular tachycardia, atrial fibrillation and atrial flutter, sometimes abruptly interrupting the arrhythmia.
   c. Testing pacemakers. The drug has been used for transient cardiac slowing to test demand pacemakers.

Dose and Duration of Effect

Edrophonium is given IV in a dose of 1 ml. (10 mg.) as a *bolus*. The onset of the drug effect is immediate, and the duration of action is usually less than 2 minutes.

Side Effects

The toxic or side effects of the drug are those of generalized parasympathetic stimulation. Tearing of the eyes, salivation, sweating, tachypnea, muscle fasciculation, abdominal cramps and even explosive diarrhea may occur.

Antidote

Atropine IV is the antidote. However, the effects of the drug would seldom last long enough to permit administration of the atropine.

NEOSTIGMINE (PROSTIGMIN)

This agent also inhibits cholinesterase, thus enhancing acetylcholine effect. The general effects are the same as those of edrophonium (Tensilon), and the dose is

0.25–0.5 mg. IV or subcutaneously. The onset of action occurs much later than that for edrophonium, and the duration of action is much longer. For these reasons, the drug has limited application in the diagnosis and treatment of cardiac arrhythmias. The side effects and antidote are the same as for edrophonium.

The Sympathetic Nervous System

INTRODUCTION

1. See Autonomic Nervous System in Chapter 2.
2. See Cardiogenic Shock, Chapter 5.

When considering drugs which affect the autonomic sympathetic nervous system it is pertinent to review the section on autonomic nervous system, particularly the sympathetic division of the autonomic nervous system. The difference between alpha adrenergic and beta adrenergic receptor effect is also an extremely important concept.

As treatment of cardiogenic shock constitutes the major use of drugs affecting the sympathetic nervous system, a review of the pathologic physiology of cardiogenic shock would also be helpful. The discussion of drugs affecting the sympathetic nervous system will ultimately be concerned with their effects on cardiogenic shock, except for propranolol.

It must be remembered that the specific effects of any drug depend on the properties of that drug, the interacting effect with other drugs, the specific disease state being treated, the ability of the body to react to and compensate for the drug, and many other factors. It is important to note that each drug may act somewhat differently in each individual patient.

ALPHA ADRENERGIC AND BETA ADRENERGIC CARDIOVASCULAR EFFECTS

The effects of alpha adrenergic and beta adrenergic stimulation have been discussed in Chapter 2. The direct cardiovascular effects are shown in Table 6. Briefly, the effects of various classes of sympathetic effective drugs are given here.

1. *Alpha and betamimetics* bring about the effects of stimulation of both receptor groups of the sympathetic nervous system, depending on the specific drug involved and the ability of the body to compensate for the effects of the drug.
2. *Alphamimetics* have vasoconstrictor action on arteries and veins. Alpha adrenergic stimulating agents cause an elevation in blood pressure, a slowing of heart rate and an increase in venous pooling.
3. *Betamimetics* have vasodilator action on arteries and veins and inotropic effects on the heart. These agents also cause a fall in blood pressure (except in some patients with shock), an increase in heart rate and a decrease in venous pooling.
4. *Alpha-blocking (alphalytic) agents* cause betamimetic peripheral vascular action by suppression of the alpha effects. Effective on both arteriolar and venular sides of the microcirculation.
5. *Beta-blocking (betalytic) agents* cause disappearance of inotropic heart effects of the beta adrenergic system. They permit predominance of alpha adrenergic effects on peripheral vascular system.

Sympathomimetic Amines

Table 7 presents a listing of the drugs affecting the sympathetic division of the autonomic nervous system, which are pertinent to acute coronary care. These drugs are used predominantly in the therapy of cardiogenic shock.

1. See discussion of catecholamines in Chapter 2.
2. See section, Autonomic Nervous System, in Chapter 2.
3. See discussion of alpha and beta adrenergic effects in Chapter 2.
4. See Chapter 5, Cardiogenic Shock.

DISCUSSION

Adrenergic-stimulating agents are essentially all sympathomimetic amines (except for angiotensin). The term "vasopressor" is used synonymously with "sympathomimetic amine" and includes both betamimetic and alphamimetic agents. These synthetic sympathomimetic compounds fall into 2 general categories.[126,133]

1. Those which combine directly with receptors, simulating the action of norepinephrine.

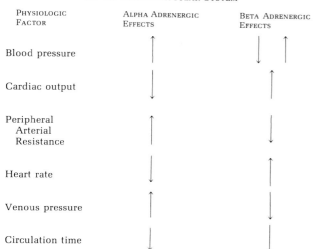

TABLE 6.—EFFECTS OF ALPHA AND BETA ADRENERGIC STIMULATION ON THE CARDIOVASCULAR SYSTEM

PHYSIOLOGIC FACTOR	ALPHA ADRENERGIC EFFECTS	BETA ADRENERGIC EFFECTS
Blood pressure	↑	↓ ↑
Cardiac output	↓	↑
Peripheral Arterial Resistance	↑	↓
Heart rate	↓	↑
Venous pressure	↑	↓
Circulation time	↓	↓

2. Those which act indirectly by liberating norepinephrine from tissue stores (metaraminol is the only one we will consider here). This second group is characterized by tachyphylaxis and referred to as norepinephrine-liberating agents.

Most sympathomimetic drugs influence both alpha and beta receptors, but the ratio of the alpha to beta activity varies tremendously between drugs. There are drugs with almost pure alpha activity and drugs with almost pure beta activity.[7] Apparently the phenylic hydroxyl groups are important for beta activity, and the amino group is important for alpha receptor stimulation.[161]

Drugs will be presented in the order in which they appear in Table 7.

NOREPINEPHRINE (LEVOPHED)*

Description

Norepinephrine is a catecholamine, a sympathomimetic amine and the naturally occurring neurotransmitter at the most peripheral synapse of the sympathetic nervous system. It is the drug (levarterenol) most commonly used to treat cardiogenic shock (see Chapter 5).

The drug, packaged commercially as Levophed, has both alpha and beta adrenergic properties, although alpha adrenergic stimulating effects predominate in the treatment of cardiogenic shock.

Action

Norepinephrine's action is essentially that of sympathetic stimulation, the alpha or beta predominance depending on the dose administered. The drug is chiefly betamimetic in effect in small doses and alphamimetic in larger doses. In excess doses it stimulates both alpha and beta receptors. The effects of norepinephrine and epinephrine are qualitatively similar though quantitatively different (a general property shared by all sympathomimetic drugs to some degree), and the 2 drugs have been extensively compared elsewhere.[7]

Specific Pharmacologic Effects

The following are properties of IV infusion of levarterenol.

1. Systolic and diastolic pressures and usually pulse pressures are increased.
2. Cardiac output is unchanged or decreased.

TABLE 7.—DRUGS AFFECTING THE SYMPATHETIC NERVOUS SYSTEM

DRUG	Alpha and Beta Stim.	Alpha Stim.	Alpha Block	Beta Stim.	COMMENT
Norepinephrine (Levophed)	*	+ + + +		+	Catecholamine, sympathomimetic amine
Epinephrine (Adrenalin)	*	+ +		+ + +	Catecholamine, sympathomimetic amine
Isoproterenol (Isuprel)				+ + + +	Catecholamine, sympathomimetic amine, betamimetic
Metaraminol (Aramine)	*	+ + + +		+	Norepinephrine-releasing drug, sympathomimetic amine
Mephentermine (Wyamine)		Very slight		+ +	Sympathomimetic amine
3-Hydroxy-tyramine (Dopamine)	*		Selective blocking		Research drug at present— precursor of norepinephrine
Methoxamine (Vasoxyl)		+ + +			Sympathomimetic amine, alphamimetic
Phenylephrine (Neo-Synephrine)	*	+ + +		+	Sympathomimetic amine
Angiotensin (Hypertensin)		*			NON-sympathomimetic drug, alphamimetic effect
Phenoxybenzamine (Dibenzyline)			*		Direct acting; alpha adrenergic blockade
Phentolamine (Regitine)			*		Direct acting; alpha adrenergic blockade
Glucocortico-steroids			*		Mechanism of action not well understood, pharmacologic doses necessary
Chlorpromazine (Thorazine)			*		Mechanism of action not well understood
Propranolol (Inderal)					Direct acting; beta blocking agent, antiarrhythmic drug

*Drug effects at this site.
There are excellent charts in the literature concerning the sympathomimetic amines.[7,133]

*References: 1, 7, 14, 25, 71, 98, 123, 133, 183.

3. Compensatory vagal reflex activity slows the heart, overcoming the direct cardioacceleration action of the drug. Thus:
4. The stroke volume is increased.
5. Total peripheral resistance is raised, with increases in most vascular beds.
   a. Blood flow is reduced through kidney, brain, liver and usually skeletal muscle.
   b. Glomerular filtration rate is maintained unless the decrease in renal blood flow is marked.
   c. There is constriction of mesenteric vessels, and splanchnic and hepatic blood flow is decreased.
   d. With reduced cerebral blood flow there is a fall in cerebral oxygen consumption.
   e. Coronary flow is substantially increased, due to coronary artery dilatation and elevated blood pressure.[7]
6. Increased force of myocardial contraction occurs.
7. Alpha-blocking agents abolish the pressor effects.
8. Circulating blood volume is decreased by loss of fluid to extracellular space via postcapillary vasoconstriction.
9. Arrhythmias have been observed.
10. The drug causes hyperglycemia.
11. Respiratory minute volume is slightly increased.
12. The drug acts on vascular smooth muscle.
13. It acts on cardiac muscle through a cellular receptor mechanism, causing positive inotropic and chronotropic effects of the heart (increased contractile force and heart rate).[133]

Interaction with Other Drugs

1. Reserpine may potentiate the effects of norepinephrine.
2. Phenothiazines (e.g., chlorpromazine) inhibits uptake of norepinephrine into cardiac storage sites. There are no effects on endogenous norepinephrine in the central nervous or vascular systems.[127]
3. Antidepressants (imipramine, desipramine, amitriptyline) inhibit uptake of norepinephrine into cardiac stores without affecting other endogenous stores.[127]

Metabolism

1. See Catecholamines in Chapter 2.
2. The drug is metabolized in the norepinephrine and epinephrine metabolic cycle. Less than 5% of an administered dose is excreted unchanged.

Indications

The prime use of this drug is in the treatment of cardiogenic shock.

Contraindications

Basically, all conditions other than cardiogenic shock are contraindications for use of the drug.

Dosage

The drug is administered only by IV infusion. It is available in 4 ml. ampules of levarterenol bitartrate injection, U.S.P. (norepinephrine) (equal to 4 mg. of active base and 8 mg. of bitartrate salt).

One ampule (4 ml.) is diluted in 1,000 ml. of solution to give a solution containing 4 μg. of levarterenol base per milliliter. Less dilute infusions may be used if large volumes of fluid are undesirable.

Some clinicians use a cardiovascular response test dose of 0.1–0.2 μg./kg. of body weight to determine individual response to the drug. The infusion is then adjusted to obtain the desired pressor response (titrated). Normally the infusion of 2–4 μg. of base/minute (0.5–1.0 ml./minute) is adequate. The pressor response to the drug can be readily controlled since it disappears within 1 or 2 minutes after the infusion is stopped. The infusion must be administered cautiously and under close observation.

Toxic and Side Effects

Untoward effects of norepinephrine (levarterenol, Levophed) are similar to those of epinephrine, but are usually minimal and less common. They are:
1. Anxiety.
2. Respiratory difficulty.
3. Awareness of the slow, foreceful heart beat.
4. Transient headache.
5. Severe hypertension, seen with overdoses, causing violent headache, photophobia, retrosternal and pharyngeal pain, pallor, intense sweating and vomiting.
6. There is a significant risk of cardiac arrhythmias.
7. If extravasation occurs at the site of IV injection, necrosis and sloughing may occur. This reaction may be prevented by local infiltration of 5 mg. of phentolamine (Regitine).

EPINEPHRINE (ADRENALIN)

Epinephrine is used in acute coronary care for cardiopulmonary resuscitation. Pharmacology of the drug is well described elsewhere,[7] and dosage is described under cardiopulmonary resuscitation (Chapter 10). This drug is used in dire emergency situations in an unconscious patient, and the side effects and toxicity will therefore not be discussed. The drug has both alpha and beta adrenergic stimulating effects.

ISOPROTERENOL (ISUPREL)

See Chapter 9 for detailed discussion of the drug.

METARAMINOL (ARAMINE)

1. See Chapter 5 for dosage in cardiogenic shock.
2. Metaraminol is a norepinephrine-releasing (liberat-

ing) drug; it acts by replacing norepinephrine in its usual storage sites and freeing the norepinephrine for its general sympathetic stimulation action previously described. The actions, therefore, are actually those of norepinephrine. Metaraminol is much less potent than norepinephrine on a milligram basis. Metaraminol has been noted to augment myocardial contraction, increase cardiac output, increase ventricular work, increase aortic pressure and coronary flow, whereas left atrial pressure may fall.[71]

Dosage

The drug is available in 1 ml. ampules and 10 ml. vials (10 mg./ml.). Metaraminol may be given by subcutaneous injection in doses of 2–10 mg.; in doses of 2–10 mg. IM; or in doses of 25–100 mg. IV in 500 to 1,000 ml. 5% D/W by infusion. Metaraminol demonstrates tachyphylaxis.

MEPHENTERMINE (WYAMINE)

Pharmacophysiology

Mephentermine is a sympathomimetic drug which has predominantly beta adrenergic stimulating action. Alpha receptor activity of the drug is relatively weak, though weak alpha receptor activity has been shown.[7] For all practical purposes in considering the drug in acute coronary care it is considered a betamimetic drug.[42] The drug causes fall in blood pressure in both normal patients and in patients in cardiogenic shock, but it increases cardiac index and systemic blood flow by its action on the myocardium and the venous circuit. The drug is particularly strong on the venous circuit, causing an increase in venous return through its beta adrenergic effect on the postcapillary venular tone.[42] Mephentermine is a direct-acting sympathomimetic drug.[126]

Dosage

The duration of pressor effects is prolonged, lasting 30–60 minutes after subcutaneous doses and up to 4 hours after IM doses. Mephentermine may be given in doses of 10–30 mg. IM. By the IV route 5–20 mg. may be given by injection, or 35–70 mg. may be added to 500 ml. 5% D/W and given by infusion.

3-HYDROXYTYRAMINE (DOPAMINE)

1. A research drug at present.
2. This drug has not had a great deal of published study to date.

Pharmacophysiology

Dopamine resembles norepinephrine and is a precursor in the natural metabolic formation of that chemi-

cal. (See Catecholamines in Chapter 2.) Dopamine resembles other sympathomimetic amines in possessing beta adrenergic cardiac-stimulating activity, but in addition it produces vasodilatation of the renal and splanchnic vascular beds selectively.[168,180]

The drug has chiefly a beta adrenergic inotropic action. It also has a slight alpha peripheral vasoconstriction action, with apparent selective blockade of peripheral vasoconstriction effects on the coronary, renal and mesenteric arteries (selective alpha blockade).

The drug appears to have an almost ideal combination of alpha and beta adrenergic activity. However, it has not been adequately investigated as yet.

Dosage

Beginning doses of 0.5 μg./kg./minute would seem indicated, with doses as high as 10 μg./kg./minute having been administered for fairly long periods.[180] It is possible that the incidence of arrhythmias with this agent is lower than it is with norepinephrine or metaraminol. Dopamine appears to release norepinephrine from storage sites.[126]

METHOXAMINE (VASOXYL)

The pharmacologic effects are almost exclusively those of alpha receptor stimulation. This drug causes increase in blood pressure due entirely to vasoconstriction. Vasoxyl has virtually no stimulant action on the heart and lacks beta receptor action on smooth muscle.[7,42,75] There is some evidence that it may depress cardiac activity despite an increase in blood pressure.[75]

Methoxamine is available in 1 ml. ampules (20 mg./ml.). The drug is given IM in a dose of 10–15 mg. and IV by adding 50 mg. to 500 ml. of 5% D/W and given by infusion.

The drug is seldom used in cardiogenic shock.

PHENYLEPHRINE (NEO-SYNEPHRINE)

Phenylephrine is a powerful alpha receptor stimulant with little effect on the beta receptors of the heart. Clinical applications of the drug depend on alpha receptor activity. This drug has essentially no place in acute coronary care.

Angiotensin (Hypertensin)

This drug is a nonsympathomimetic drug, infrequently used in acute coronary care. The actions depend on its alpha receptor stimulation. The drug may be administered in a dose of 2.5–7.5 mg. in 500 ml. 5% D/W at a rate of 3–10 μg./minute or more rapidly if required.

Alpha Adrenergic Blocking Agents

Alpha adrenergic agents affect the sympathetic nervous system by causing blockade of the alpha receptors.

Phenoxybenzamine (POB, Dibenzyline)

Description

Phenoxybenzamine is a haloalkylamine. Members of this series produce a prolonged blockade of alpha adrenergic receptors.

Actions

1. Phenoxybenzamine (POB) is used at present by some clinicians in the treatment of the shock syndrome. Therefore, discussion of the effects of this drug will relate to this particular use. The drug is not as yet approved by the Food and Drug Administration for this purpose.
2. POB effectively prevents responses to adrenergic stimuli that are mediated by alpha receptors. The drug:
   a. Inhibits responses to circulating catecholamines better than responses of those catecholamines released locally at nerve endings.
   b. Does not alter those effects mediated by beta adrenergic receptors.
3. POB does not have direct cardiac effects, but effects are indirectly exerted. Total peripheral resistance is decreased. This decreases arterial blood pressure and thus affects cardiac output.
4. The improved urine flow after POB in cardiogenic shock is partially due to improved splanchnic and renal flow, but part may be due to a central nervous system mechanism.
5. In experimental animals POB has been seen to improve pulmonary perfusion.
6. POB is a moderately potent antihistamine and antiserotonin. These two substances play an as yet undetermined role in cardiogenic shock.
7. POB effectively inhibits cardiac arrhythmias induced by sympathomimetic amines in man. This is in contrast to the drug's lack of effect on physiologic responses of the myocardium.
8. POB can stimulate the central nervous system to cause nausea, vomiting, hyperventilation, motor excitability and even convulsions when it is injected rapidly IV in relatively large doses. These effects are unrelated to the alpha adrenergic blockade produced by the agent.

Metabolism

The metabolic fate of POB is poorly understood. Over 50% of radioactive POB is excreted in 12 hours and over 80% in 24 hours, but small amounts remain in various tissues for at least a week.

Indications

Therapy of cardiogenic shock. It is a research drug for this use.

Contraindication

Lack of ability to monitor central venous pressure and provide volume expansion for the increased capacitance that will occur with the alpha adrenergic blockade.

Dosage and Administration

1. For practical purposes, in acute coronary care POB is given only by the IV route.
2. The commonest dosage is 1 mg./kg. diluted in 250–500 ml. of 5% D/W and infused over a period of at least 1 hour and preferably 2–4 hours.
   a. The drug acts within minutes to decrease peripheral resistance.[130]
   b. The peak effect is probably reached in 1 hour. After a single dose, a progressively decreasing, but still significant, blockade persists for at least 3–4 days.
   c. Cumulative effect occurs with daily administration, for at least 3–4 days.
   d. The central venous pressure (CVP) is maintained at 10–12 cm. water before, during and for 24 hours after the administration of POB. The choice of volume expander depends on the hematocrit value.

Toxic Effects

1. Toxic effects are largely extensions of the desired blockade of alpha adrenergic receptors, namely, loss of vasomotor control with the occurrence of severe hypotension.
2. Since alpha adrenergic blockade increases capacitance and POB induces loss of arteriolar and venular tone, thus reducing capillary hydrostatic pressure and enlarging the venular capacitance, the following precautions must be observed when POB is used in the therapy of shock.
   a. Administration of POB in shock must be coupled with adequate volume replacement.
   b. Volume deficits may be corrected with reasonable accuracy by monitoring central venous pressure during fluid replacement.[133]
3. Moderate hypercapnia (increased CO_2), which normally leaves the blood pressure unaltered or causes a slight rise, can produce marked hypotension after POB blockade, as can doses of analgesics such as morphine or meperidine.
4. Specific liver, kidney or bone-marrow damage has not been observed; however, POB is still undergoing clinical investigation and should be used with caution.

Phentolamine (Regitine)

Description

Phentolamine is an imidazoline derivative chemically.

Action

Note: There are numerous effects other than alpha adrenergic blockade—some undesirable.

1. Phentolamine produces moderately effective, competitive alpha adrenergic blockade, which is relatively transient. Other physiologic actions are also produced.
2. The drug has direct effects on vascular smooth muscle, causing vasodilatation in the systemic and pulmonary vascular systems.
3. It does not inhibit chronotropic or inotropic responses of myocardium to adrenergic stimuli, and it is itself an effective myocardial stimulant.
4. Cardiac stimulation is commonly produced by therapeutic doses in man and is a prominent symptom of overdosage. There may be associated arrhythmias.
5. The drug does not effectively inhibit the relaxant effects of epinephrine on the gastrointestinal musculature, and itself induces hyperperistalsis and diarrhea. This motor response is blocked by atropine. Gastric secretion is stimulated by the drug.

Metabolism

Exact metabolism of the drug is undetermined. However, the drug is rapidly excreted by the kidney. It is excreted largely unchanged by the renal tubules.

Indications

1. Phentolamine in combination with norepinephrine has been suggested to be superior to norepinephrine alone in the treatment of cardiogenic shock.
2. Phentolamine is used as a test for pheochromocytoma.
3. Phentolamine may be infiltrated locally if norepinephrine has extravasated out of the vein in order to prevent the necrosis and sloughing of tissue frequently caused by norepinephrine under these conditions.

Contraindications

1. As for phenoxybenzamine.
2. In situations in which toxicity symptoms would be undesirable.
3. *Note:* In the small doses used, the likelihood of complications is not great.

Dosage and Administration

Phentolamine comes in 5 mg. ampules. In therapy of cardiogenic shock, 5 mg. may be added to 1,000 ml. 5% D/W containing the appropriate amount of norepinephrine, and this combination used.

Toxicity

Toxicity is attributable to cardiac and gastrointestinal stimulation. Cardiac stimulation can cause alarming tachycardia, cardiac arrhythmias and anginal pain after parenteral administration (undesirable effect of higher doses). Gastrointestinal stimulation may result in abdominal pain, nausea, vomiting and diarrhea, and exacerbation of peptic ulcer.

It has been suggested that this drug be used with caution in coronary artery disease. It would seem therefore that the drug is too toxic to use alone or in higher doses in the acute coronary care setting.

OTHER ANTIADRENERGIC AGENTS

The effects of other antiadrenergic agents, such as guanethidine (Ismelin) and bretylium; of other agents which affect catecholamine levels of the tissue, such as reserpine, rauwolfia and methyldopa, as well as of the ganglionic blocking agents, are adequately set forth in many other reference sources.

GLUCOCORTICOSTEROIDS

1. These agents, when given in *pharmacologic* doses, have alpha adrenergic effects produced by as yet undetermined mechanisms.
2. See Treatment of Cardiogenic Shock, Chapter 5, and Steroids, Chapter 16.

CHLORPROMAZINE (THORAZINE)

Description

Chlorpromazine is one of the phenothiazine derivatives and has an alpha adrenergic blockade effect. It is one of the most widely used drugs in the practice of medicine today. During the past decade at least 50 million patients have received chlorpromazine and more than 10,000 publications have dealt with its actions.[7] The drug has had essentially all of its use in the psychotherapeutic field.

Adequate presentations of the general pharmacology may be found in other sources.

Chlorpromazine has been used in the treatment of shock as an alpha adrenergic blocking agent and for its other physiologic effects. Our discussion will be limited to this aspect of the drug's use.

Action

1. Chlorpromazine has been found to be an alpha adrenergic blocking agent, with the exact mechanism of alpha blockade not well defined.
2. Its multiple mechanisms of action on the central and autonomic nervous systems render it potentially useful in the treatment of shock. Among these are the following:[133]
   a. Ability to decrease the electrical excitability of

the limbic cortex and thalamocortical radiations without directly affecting sensory or motor pathways, producing tranquilizing effects.

b. Ability to inhibit hypothalamic mechanisms governing thermoregulation and vasomotor response, and possibly to suppress the action of adrenergic amines in the brain.

c. Ability to inhibit the effects of adrenergic amines on vascular smooth muscle in pulmonary as well as muscular and cutaneous vascular beds (alpha blockade).

d. An effect on oxidative metabolism in cells affording some degree of protection of ischemic tissue from hypoxia.

e. No consistent effects on heart rate, contractile force or stroke volume.

f. It may inhibit cardiac uptake of norepinephrine.[127]

Metabolism

The metabolic pathways of chlorpromazine are complex.[7]

Dosage and Administration

As used in acute coronary care in the treatment of cardiogenic shock (Chapter 5), chlorpromazine is usually administered IV in a dose of 1 mg./kg. and given over a 10–15 minute period. Chlorpromazine does not produce the dramatic decreases in vascular capacitance seen with phenoxybenzamine, because its alpha-blocking effects are not nearly as strong. However, central venous monitoring and treatment with volume expanders must be used, as with phenoxybenzamine.[135]

PROPRANOLOL (INDERAL)

1. See section on Propranolol, Chapter 9.
2. A beta adrenergic blockade agent.

CHAPTER 16

Other Therapeutic Agents

Cathartics

DEFINITION

Cathartics are drugs that promote defecation.

INDICATIONS

The necessity to prevent constipation has been discussed previously in section on Bowel Care and Control (Chapter 8). This section deals only with the various cathartics and their action. There are many different drugs and drug combinations utilized to stimulate defecation. No attempt will be made here to list these by their trade names. The specific drug or drugs present in any given cathartic preparation may be easily found in other sources.[7]

Cathartics are definitely indicated in many instances for therapy of patients in the acute coronary care unit.

CLASSIFICATION

Cathartics are sometimes classified according to intensity of effect (laxatives, purgatives and drastics), according to the site of action or by the latency of their cathartic effect. The most useful method of classification for our purposes is based upon the mechanism of action (see Table 8).

1. Stimulant cathartics
   a. Anthraquinone derivatives (mainly large bowel stimulation).
      1) Cascara sagrada and senna.
      2) Danthron.
   b. Phenolphthalein (predominant effect on colon; small intestinal activity may also be increased).
      1) Acetphenolisatin, derivative of phenolphthalein used in Europe.
   c. Bisacodyl (more active on the large bowel).
      1) Sometimes called a contact cathartic.
      2) Available in rectal suppositories.
   d. Castor oil. Unlike other stimulant cathartics, this compound stimulates the *small intestine.*

2. Saline cathartics
   a. Magnesium salts.
      1) Magnesium sulfate (Epsom salt).
      2) Milk of magnesia (aqueous suspension of magnesium hydroxide).
      3) Magnesium citrate.
   b. Sodium salts.
      1) Sodium sulfate.
      2) Sodium phosphate (dibasic sodium phosphate).
   c. Potassium salts.
      1) Potassium *sodium* tartrate. Usually sodium bicarbonate and tartaric acid are mixed and administered just after effervescence begins to subside.
      2) Potassium bitartrate (cream of tartar).

3. Bulk-forming cathartics
   a. Various natural and semisynthetic polysaccharides and cellulose derivatives.
      1) Methylcellulose and sodium carboxymethyl-cellulose.
      2) Plantago seed (psyllium seed).
      3) Agar and tragacanth.
      4) Bran.

TABLE 8.—CLASSIFICATION AND MECHANISM OF ACTION OF CATHARTICS

CLASS OF CATHARTIC	MECHANISM OF ACTION	EFFECT ON PERISTALSIS	FORMS BULK
Stimulant (irritant)	Increases motor activity of intestinal tract (direct)	Direct stimulation	
Saline	The salts are *slowly* absorbed from digestive tract, and water is retained in the intestinal lumen by osmosis—effectively increasing intestinal bulk	Indirectly increases	X
Bulk-forming	Indigestible water-absorbing colloids increase bulk in intestinal lumen; may soften feces	Indirectly increases	X
Lubricant	Facilitates defecation by softening and lubricating the feces; no other action		

4. Lubricant cathartics

  a. Mineral oil. This acts as a lipid solvent and may interfere with absorption of essential fat-soluble substances, particularly vitamins A, D and K.

  b. Dioctyl sodium sulfosuccinate, an anionic surface-active agent.

Electrotrophic Drugs

In considering electrolytes and drugs which affect electrolytes (electrotrophic drugs), it must be remembered that the fund of information concerning electrolyte influences, in particular on the cardiovascular system, is increasing almost daily. An attempt to present some of this information, admittedly fragmentary in nature, follows and refers to the specific subject under consideration.

EFFECTS OF IONIC CHANGES ON CARDIAC STATUS

1. Electrolyte ions which *increase* irritability and contractility of the heart are:
   sodium (Na^+), calcium (Ca^{++}) and hydroxy (OH^-).
2. Electrolyte ions which *decrease* irritability and contractility of the heart are:
   potassium (K^+), magnesium (Mg^{++}) and
   hydrogen (H^+).
3. Discussion: The cardiovascular changes brought about by electrolyte ionic changes and the administration of electrolyte therapy can be understood with reference to the effects of the above ions and changes from their normal status in the body, as related to their cardiac effect.

DRUGS WHICH AFFECT BODY ELECTROLYTES

1. Drugs for general electrolyte therapy.
     a. Maintenance solutions.
     b. Therapeutic solutions to combat acidosis and alkalosis, whatever the cause.
     c. Infusions of specific electrolyte solutions, e.g., potassium chloride, sodium bicarbonate, sodium lactate, etc.
     d. Oral ingestion of electrolytes in various forms.
2. Digitalis preparations (cardiac glycosides).
3. Diuretics.
4. Chelating agents (EDTA).

ELECTROLYTES AND DRUGS USED IN DIGITALIS INTOXICATION

1. Potassium salts are given for digitalis intoxication, either by IV infusion of a solution of potassium chloride (see Digitalis Intoxication in Chapter 12), or by oral ingestion of potassium salts. Gluconate and other salts of potassium are used when the hydrogen and chloride ion levels have not been affected.

2. Ethylenediamine tetra-acetate (EDTA) has been utilized, but the toxic effects are potentially so great with this agent that it is probably not advisable in a patient suffering acute myocardial infarction.
     a. EDTA acts by chelating calcium, which is a myocardial irritant, and thereby enhancing the reciprocal effect of the potassium which is present.

ELECTROLYTES FOR DIURETIC TOXICITY

1. Usually diuretic effect and digitalis presence in the body combine to cause a more hazardous situation than would result from either drug alone.
2. Potassium salts are administered to correct this situation, either orally or by infusion of potassium chloride.
     a. When administered orally, potassium salts other than chloride are sometimes used.
     b. In the presence of hypochloremic alkalosis—caused by loss of hydrogen and chloride ions—when the newer, more potent diuretics cause profuse diuresis, potassium *chloride* therapy is specifically utilized, whether given IV or orally.

ELECTROLYTES FOR CARDIAC RESUSCITATION

1. With cardiac resuscitation, electrolyte ions are injected (either by IV or intracardiac route) to cause a cardiac irritating (stimulating) effect in order to make the myocardium more susceptible to defibrillation. These are calcium ion solutions as follows:
     a. Calcium chloride, 10 ml. of 10% solution.
     b. Calcium gluconate, 10 ml. of 10% solution.

ELECTROLYTES TO CORRECT ACIDOSIS

1. Acidosis occurs with tissue hypoxia. Metabolic acidosis occurs rapidly in the presence of profound cardiogenic shock or in the presence of cardiac arrest. Any condition which temporarily decreases the cardiac output significantly, causing tissue hypoxia, will produce acidosis. Cardiac arrest is the most severe form of decreased cardiac output.
2. Metabolic acidosis is usually correlated with a tendency to arrhythmias of the death-producing types, even if no such arrhythmia existed prior to the metabolic acidosis.
3. Sodium bicarbonate in doses of approximately 40 mEq. (3.36 Gm.) is injected IV every 8–10 minutes in the presence of "cardiac arrest." A 5% solution of sodium bicarbonate may also be used and is infused at a rate of about 75 ml. every 5 minutes.
4. Molar sodium lactate has been used to combat acidosis, particularly when AV block is present and the block is being potentiated by increased serum potassium levels.

THAM

The drug THAM has been used as an organic buffered material to combat acidosis when great care must be taken with sodium-containing solutions. It is difficult and time consuming to use.

Potassium-Glucose-Insulin

These solutions have been utilized for "polarizing" therapy in the prophylaxis of arrhythmias in acute myocardial infarction, and more specifically in the therapy of AV block arrhythmias. The value of such therapy is debated and has not as yet been definitely determined.

Dextran 40 (LMD, Rheomacrodex)

Description

Dextran 40[10,217] is a preparation of low molecular weight dextran, having an average molecular weight of approximately 40,000. It is also referred to as low viscosity dextran, in contrast to dextran 75 (also known as clinical dextran) which has an average molecular weight of 75,000. Dextran 40 is a polysaccharide material made up of molecules with a weight of 10,000 to 90,000, averaging 40,000, in which 90% of the cross-linkages of the polysaccharide are of the 1, 6 glucosidic, straight-chain type.

Action on Microcirculation

1. **Expands volume.** Dextran 40 increases circulatory volume directly by infusion and indirectly by osmotic attraction of extravascular interstitial fluid (extracellular fluid outside the vascular system).
2. **Maintains charges.** It helps maintain the electronegative charge on the surface of red blood cells, thus causing the red blood cells to be mutually repellent and helping to prevent sludging and aggregation of red cells.
3. **Coats cells.** It provides a coating effect to the red blood cells and platelets, improving the flow characteristics of blood in the microcirculation.
4. **Improves suspension.** It improves the suspension stability of the blood, so that formed elements have less tendency to settle out, thus enhancing flow in microcirculation.
5. **Reduces viscosity.** As a result of hemodilution and lowered hematocrit as well as attraction of extracellular fluid, the viscosity of the blood is lowered, further promoting improved microcirculation.

Metabolism and Excretion

1. Plasma concentration of dextran 40 varies with the rate of infusion, the total amount administered and the disappearance from the plasma.
2. During infusion, dextran 40 is evenly distributed in the vascular system.
3. After infusion, the plasma concentration falls rapidly in the first hour and thereafter more slowly.
4. The higher molecular fractions remain in the vascular system longer than small molecules which are excreted by the kidney.
5. Following infusion (in patients with normal blood volume), 50% is excreted within 3 hours, 60% within 6 hours and 75% within 24 hours.
6. A portion of dextran 40 is excreted into the gastrointestinal tract and eliminated in the feces.
7. Reabsorption of dextran by renal tubules is negligible.
8. Unexcreted molecules of dextran 40 diffuse into the extravascular compartment and are temporarily taken up by the reticuloendothelial system.
9. Some of the molecules are then returned to the intravascular compartment from the reticuloendothelial system via the lymphatics.
10. Dextran is slowly degraded to glucose by the enzyme dextranase.

Indications

Since we are here predominantly concerned with the use of dextran 40 in cardiogenic shock, our discussion will be relevant to that use only. Dextran has been reported useful in other types of shock and has been used following pulmonary embolus.

1. Dextran 40 has been used by clinicians in the treatment of cardiogenic shock in conjunction with alpha adrenergic blockade types of therapy and with beta adrenergic stimulation therapy. In the treatment of shock it is used for its effect on the *microcirculation* (see Chapter 5, Cardiogenic Shock).
2. **Effects in shock.** Note that the results listed below are not limited to the *CARDIOGENIC* type of shock.
   a. Dextran 40 produces significant increase in blood volume, central venous pressure, cardiac output, stroke volume and blood pressure and quickly restores the reduced intravascular volume.
   b. It produces an increase in cardiac index up to 150% of control values.
   c. Urinary output is increased.
   d. It reduces blood viscosity and peripheral resistance, prevents or lessens intravascular blood sludging and cell aggregation and improves the peripheral blood flow in the microcirculation with a release of sequestered cells, thereby increasing venous blood return to the heart.

Contraindications

1. Dextran 40 is contraindicated in the presence of thrombocytopenia and hypofibrinogenemia and in renal disease with severe oliguria or anuria.
2. **Precautions**
   a. Dosage exceeding those recommended may cause prolongation of bleeding time.

1) In recommended dosage dextran 40 has no significant effect on the coagulation of blood outside the microcirculation.
    b. Dextrans of molecular weight higher than that of dextran 40 may produce erythrocyte aggregation and interfere with blood typing and cross-matching. Dextran 40 is said not to interfere with these procedures.

3. **Warnings**
    a. Dextran 40 is a hypertonic colloid-like solution. It attracts water from the extravascular space. This shift of fluid should be considered if the drug is used in poorly hydrated patients. Additional fluid therapy will be needed in poorly hydrated patients.
    b. If dextran 40 is given in excess, vascular overload with the occurrence of pulmonary edema may occur. This possibility may be avoided by careful central venous pressure (CVP) monitoring.

Dosage and Administration

1. The basic principle is to give the minimum needed to restore blood flow.
2. It is suggested that total dosage should not exceed 20 ml./kg. during the first 24 hours.
    a. The first 10 ml./kg. may be infused as rapidly as necessary to effect improvement.
    b. The second 10 ml./kg., if needed, should be infused more slowly.
    c. If therapy is continued beyond 24 hours, subsequent dosage should not exceed 10 ml./kg./day.
3. It is strongly recommended that central venous pressure be monitored frequently during infusion. Proponents of use of alpha adrenergic blocking agents with dextran or other volume expanders suggest that central venous pressure monitoring is mandatory in this type of therapy for shock.

Toxicity

1. Toxicity may result from misuse of dextran 40; see above.
2. Dextran 40 has been reported to be *nephrotonic*; however, renal failure has been reported to occur after its use. It may be questionable whether renal failure was secondary to dextran 40 or to the primary condition requiring its use.
3. Renal tubular vacuolation has been found following dextran 40 administration in animals and man. This appears to be reversible and to be a consequence of high urine concentration of the drug. Its exact clinical significance is presently unknown.
4. Antigenic reactions are few. Antigenicity of dextrans is directly related to the degree of branching chains. Dextran 40 has a low degree of branching and is relatively free of antigenic effect. However, the following should be noted:

    a. A few individuals have had mild urticarial reactions.
    b. In rare instances, more severe reactions of generalized urticaria, tightness of the chest, wheezing, hypotension and nausea and vomiting may occur.
    c. Signs and symptoms of adverse systemic reactions may be relieved by parenteral administration of antihistamines or epinephrine.
    d. When dextran 40 is used in recommended dosage, with proper monitoring, the likelihood of untoward effects is minimized.

Steroids

Steroids have been utilized for several specific situations in the therapy of various aspects of acute myocardial infarction. That steroid therapy is not consistently used in these situations attests to the fact that, whether they are of value under these circumstances is not fully determined.

Specific Pharmacology

The specifics of the pharmacology are complex and have been well investigated. No attempt will be made here to present any appreciable detail of the pharmacology of the various glucocorticosteroids; excellent coverage may be found in numerous other sources.[7,10]

Major Actions

The major actions of steroids in cardiogenic shock therapy will be presented as an example of the general beneficial effects of steroid therapy in situations associated with acute myocardial infarction. These actions are as follows[124]:
1. Alpha adrenergic blockage effect: useful in the therapy of cardiogenic shock at the pharmacologic (not physiologic) dosages used in therapy of this complication.
2. Nonspecific effects on the tissue.
3. Local action at the cellular level.
4. Protection of cells from injury by noxious stimuli via
    a. Maintenance of cell membrane integrity.
    b. Stabilization of lysozomes of the cell.
    c. With respect to cardiogenic shock, protection at the cellular level is proportionate to the concentration achieved at the cellular level.
5. Increase in cardiac output—inotropic action.
    See also specific agents in therapy of cardiogenic shock, Chapter 5.

Side Effects of Steroid Therapy (in Physiologic Doses)

1. The major side effects of steroid therapy are well known and chiefly are as follows:
    a. Delay of healing and poor healing.

b. Activation of peptic ulcer disease and occurrence of peptic ulcer disease.
c. Fluid retention. Fluid and salt retention could precipitate pulmonary edema.
d. Activation of granulomatous lesions of the lung and other organs.
e. Superimposed infection—due to inability of the usual body defenses to combat infection.
f. Steroid withdrawal (adrenal insufficiency) at termination of therapy.

2. Drugs affecting steroid therapy:
a. Antihistamines, barbiturates and diphenylhydantoin (Dilantin) have all been found to inhibit the effectiveness of steroids.

SPECIFIC USES IN PRESENCE OF ACUTE MYOCARDIAL INFARCTION

1. **Cardiogenic shock.** See Cardiogenic Shock, Chapter 5.

a. Dosages as presented in section on Steroids, Chapter 5.
b. Effectiveness is determined by concentration at the receptor site; therefore, analogues of cortisol equilibrate more rapidly between blood and tissues and maintain a higher effective level, as they do not compete with cortisol for protein-binding sites.[124]

2. **AV block.** Use of steroids in heart block is by no means accepted; however, therapy is carried out by some clinicians.[16,105,148,149]
a. Large doses, equal to 60–80 mg. prednisone, are sometimes used in the first 24 hours in the therapy of AV block.[16]

3. **Pericarditis.** Steroids have been administered by some investigators in selected instances of pericarditis.

4. **Diaphragmatic (inferior) infarcts.** Steroids have been utilized by some investigators in the therapy of this localization of acute myocardial infarction.

Representative Procedures and Protocols; Information for Physicians and Nurses

Introduction

The following procedure protocols, emergency protocols, tables and informational discussions are not intended to represent exact protocols which should necessarily be used in every institution. They are modifications of protocols and information utilized in various hospitals of various sizes and are intended as *representative examples* to provide general guidelines. The medical director of the coronary care unit and the coronary care committee, in conjunction with the nursing staff, will outline the appropriate procedures and protocols utilized on a regular basis for the various situations which arise in the coronary care unit of each institution, and they will make this information available to the coronary care unit personnel. The procedures and protocols for a given hospital will depend on the specific circumstances and possibilities for each clinical situation as they relate to the facilities and personnel of the particular institution. Therefore, individual procedures and protocols for each hospital can be compiled and standardized only on a specific basis for that institution.

It is hoped that some of the information in these representative protocols may be used in composite form to formulate procedural policies in the institutions served by those reading this manual. It is particularly anticipated that a composite type of use might be especially helpful in establishing policies for coronary care units in *smaller* hospitals.

For Emergency Situations

Coronary Care Unit—Emergency Procedure

RESPONSE TO ALARM

The nurse goes to patient's bedside in response to alarm.

1. If false alarm, nurse turns off alarm and determines the cause of the false alarm.
2. If cardiac arrest or other serious arrhythmia has occurred, the nurse will push the emergency button or otherwise summon emergency aid.
3. In cases of cardiac arrest, the nurse will determine whether the emergency is due to ventricular fibrillation or to asystole.

VENTRICULAR FIBRILLATION

If the arrest is due to ventricular fibrillation, the following will be noted:
1. The abnormal rhythm will be seen on the oscilloscope.

2. The patient will be unconscious or becoming comatose.
3. The skin will be cyanotic, moist and cool.
4. The patient may convulse.
5. The pulse will be unobtainable.

Procedure in Ventricular Fibrillation

1. The first shock of 400 watt-seconds should be given as soon as possible, either by the emergency team or by the nurse.
2. If the first is not effective, the second shock should be given within 10 seconds.
3. If a second shock is not effective, start closed chest cardiac resuscitation immediately.
4. 75 ml. of 5% sodium bicarbonate may be given every 5 minutes unless subsequent pH determination contraindicates it.
5. 50–100 mg. lidocaine (2.5–5 ml. of 2% solution) is given by IV bolus. Three or 4 minutes later, a shock

of 400 watt-seconds may be attempted again. Arterial blood samples may be drawn for pH, oxygen and hematocrit determinations.

6. If the heart still cannot be defibrillated, 0.5 ml. epinephrine, 1:1,000 solution (diluted to 5 ml.), is injected directly into the heart and an additional shock is given.

ASYSTOLE

If the arrest is due to asystole:

1. The monitor will display a straight-line pattern.
2. Patient appearance and vital signs will be the same as those noted under Ventricular Fibrillation.

Procedure in Cardiac Asystole

1. External pacing is seldom successful and wastes precious time.
2. Begin closed chest cardiac resuscitation immediately.
3. 75 ml. of 5% sodium bicarbonate is given every 5 minutes unless a subsequent pH determination contraindicates it.
4. 1 mg. Isuprel (isoproterenol) in 500 ml. of 5% D/W is started IV.
5. Levophed (norepinephrine) may be added to the IV infusion.

6. If these measures fail, an intracardiac pacing wire may be inserted directly through the chest wall into the left ventricular cavity for electrical pacing.
7. If pacing is ineffective, 0.5 ml. epinephrine, 1:1,000 solution (diluted to 5 ml.), may be given directly into the heart or Levophed given IV.

IDIOVENTRICULAR RATE OF LESS THAN 40

The patient may be alert and conscious or may show signs of increasing loss of consciousness.

Procedure when Idioventricular Rate is Less than 40

1. 1 mg. atropine may be given IV.
2. If atropine fails to increase the heart rate, Isuprel (isoproterenol) in a concentration of 1 mg. in 500 ml. of 5% D/W is given IV, using a microdrip.
3. If this is ineffective, electrical pacing may be used via a transvenous pacing electrode. Isuprel drip is continued until pacing is started.
4. Lidocaine may be necessary to suppress Isuprel ventricular irritability.

Coronary Care Unit—Emergency Procedure in Brief

VENTRICULAR FIBRILLATION	ASYSTOLE	IDIOVENTRICULAR RHYTHM WITH RATE < 40 AND SYSTOLIC BLOOD PRESSURE < 70 MM. HG
Stage I Shock, 400 ws., 10 sec. pause; repeat if ineffective CCCR	*Stage I* Begin CCCR	*Stage I* Call physician Stat; have Isuprel drip prepared
NaHCO$_3$ IV every 5 min., 75 ml. of 5%	NaHCO$_3$ IV every 5 min., 75 ml. of 5%	
Stage II Lidocaine IV, 25–100 mg., or Pronestyl, 50–250 mg. 3–4 min. after lidocaine or Pronestyl, shock of 400 ws. if VF persists	*Stage II* If above has failed, Isuprel IV, 1 mg. in 500 ml. D5W Transthoracic pacing wire	*Stage II* Atropine, 1 mg. in 10 ml. N/S IV Isuprel, 1 mg./500 ml. D5W IV.
	Adrenalin IC, 0.5 ml. 1:1,000 (5 ml. of 1:10,000)	Transvenous pacemaker
Other drugs which may be used before repeat shock, if above has failed: Adrenalin IC, 0.5 ml. 1:1,000 (5 ml. of 1:10,000) Shock of 400 ws.	Levophed IV	

Stage I: Absence of the physician
Stage II: Presence of the physician
CCCR: Closed chest cardiac resuscitation
IC: Intracardiac
ws.: Watt-seconds

TABLE 9.—EMERGENCY ROUTINE FOR CARDIAC ARRHYTHMIAS

These instructions are complementary to and do not conflict with the previously issued instructions governing nurses working in the coronary intensive care area. The usually successful procedures in the right-hand column are recommended but are left to the physician's discretion.

In all cases access to the central vascular system will be established immediately via needle or intracath and kept open with 1,000 ml. 5% D/W containing 20 mg. heparin and run at 20 drops/minute via microdrip tubing.

CONDITION	SUGGESTED MANAGEMENT To be Instituted by Nurses and Doctors Notified of Your Action	Suggestions for the Doctor
Rare PACs	None	
Frequent bigeminal or trigeminal PACs	Notify doctor (Urgent)	Digitalize, or quinidine sulfate 200 mg. q 6 hr.
Supraventricular tachycardia Atrial or AV nodal a. Simple	Notify doctor Stat ECG (12 lead)	Adequate sedation helpful Ocular or unilateral carotid pressure;
b. With 2d-degree AV block		Digitalize and repeat carotid pressure. IV glucose (5% in 500 ml.) with 40 mEq. potassium chloride and 10 units regular insulin added
Atrial flutter	Notify doctor (Urgent) Stat ECG (12 lead)	Usually digitalize: cedilanid-D in digitalizing dose of 1.6 mg. (8 ml.); give IV in divided doses—½, ¼, ¼. If urgent, may be given in a single IV injection slowly. If reversion occurs, maintain with quinidine; if not, cardiovert.
Atrial fibrillation	Notify doctor (Urgent) Stat ECG (12 lead)	If rapid ventricular rate, slow with digitalis as above. If slowing is not successful, do elective cardioversion—maintain conversion with quinidine.
Rare PVCs	None	
PVCs interrupting T-waves, salvos of 2 or more PVCs, multiform PVCs or sustained at more than 5/min.	50 mg. bolus of lidocaine (Xylocaine) in single IV injection. If arrhythmia persists, repeat 50 mg. bolus of lidocaine. If successful, maintain with IV drip delivering 1–2 mg./min. or enough to suppress recurrence. If ineffective, give procainamide (Pronestyl) IV 50 mg. every 2-3 min. until arrhythmia is abolished; don't exceed 250 mg. in 20 min. Then give oral or IM procainamide (0.5-1 Gm. q4-6 hr. orally; 0.5-1 Gm. q6 hr. IM).	
Ventricular tachycardia a. Self-terminating; brief paroxysms of 4–20 beats	Stat ECG (12 lead) Same as PVCs above	
b. Rapid and sustained	Lidocaine (Xylocaine) 50 mg. bolus; Repeat with 100 mg. if necessary; maintain as for PVCs above. If no response ⟶	Cardioversion
Ventricular fibrillation (Unconscious patient)	1. Initiate Code Blue 2. Cardiopulmonary resuscitation 3. Start NaHCO₃	Defibrillate (See cardiopulmonary Resuscitation)
Bradycardia: rate 50 or below	Notify doctor If persists over 1 hr., give atropine sulfate 0.6-1 mg. IV	Atropine gr. 1/100 IV or Isuprel linguette (10 mg.) q3 hr. or Isuprel IV drip (1.0 mg. in 500 ml. 5% D/W); titrate to 60 beats/min. Avoid producing excess premature contractions.
AV block 1st degree—PR over 0.2 sec. 2d degree—some unconducted P-waves 3d degree—AV dissociation	Notify doctor (Urgent)	1. No treatment 2. Same as bradycardia above 3. Isuprel as above; if unsuccessful, use transvenous pacemaker
Pulmonary edema (severe)	Rotating tourniquets Notify doctor (Urgent) Stat ECG (12 lead) Ethacrynic acid (Edecrin), 50 mg. in 50 ml. 5% D/W IV slowly (several minutes) or Lasix, 20 mg. IV., slowly Venesection	Digitalize as above Morphine gr. 1/6 usually most effective. Venesection
Shock	Notify doctor (Urgent) Aramine, 100 mg. in 1,000 ml. 5% D/W (1 ml. amp. contains 10 mg.). Titrate.	Aramine, 100 mg. in 1,000 ml. 5% D/W (10 ml. vial contains 100 mg.). Titrate. Levophed, 4–8 mg. in 1,000 ml. 5% D/W (4 ml. amp. contains 4 mg.). Add 5 mg. Regitine (1 ml. amp. contains 5 mg.) to this dose.

PROCEDURE AFTER RESUSCITATION

When an effective heart beat has been established, attention should be given to vital signs, fluid and electrolyte balance, indicated laboratory determinations and general care. A portable chest x-ray should be taken after all instances of cardiac resuscitation.

Recommended Steps for Cardiopulmonary Resuscitation (Applies Outside CCU Also)

1. Diagnose: Apnea, no pulse, unconsciousness.
2. Note size of pupils, observe time.
3. Initiate Emergency Cardiac Arrest Notification Procedure (Code Blue, Code 99, etc.)
4. Deliver a sharp blow with the fist to the sternal area. This may be all that is needed to restore breathing and heart action.
5. Start artificial ventilation: Clear airway, hyperextend head, close nose, give 3 or 4 puffs into patient's mouth or nose.
6. Start external cardiac massage.
   a. Bare the chest and locate lower one-third of sternum.
   b. Place heel (not palm) of hand over lower one-third of sternum, with pressure of second hand on top of first hand. Give a thrust vertically downward, moving the sternum 1½–2 in. toward the spine. Use force of one hand in children and of 2 fingers in newborn. (Proper placement of hands is essential for effective massage and to avoid complications.)
   c. Depress sternum once a second in adults. Release pressure completely after each compression, but do not raise hands from sternum.
   d. Check effectiveness (femoral or carotid pulsation and constricting pupils).
7. If alone, interrupt massage every 15–30 seconds to inflate lungs a few times.
8. Start an IV infusion with 5% sodium bicarbonate solution (75 ml. every 5 minutes) and with 100 mg. Aramine (metaraminol) or 16 mg. Levophed, as soon as possible.
9. Take an ECG to determine the type of arrest.

TYPES OF ARREST TO BE DEFIBRILLATED

1. Ventricular tachycardia.
2. Ventricular fibrillation or flutter.
   These are the only rhythms causing "cardiac arrest" which respond to the use of the defibrillator.

STEPS IN DEFIBRILLATION

Step 1. If you can defibrillate before 30–45 seconds have elapsed, do so without other resuscitative procedures. If over 45 seconds, resuscitate.
   a. Ventricular tachycardia: Use synchronized shock at 50-watt-seconds initially. Then if there is no response, increase to 100, 200 and 400 watt-seconds respectively.
   b. After applying electrode jelly to each of the electrode paddles, position one paddle in the area of the second intercostal space, along the right sternal border, and position the other paddle in the 5th or 6th interspace, at the apex of the heart. BE SURE THAT NO ONE IS TOUCHING THE PATIENT OR THE BED, AND THAT THE PATIENT CABLE OF THE ELECTROCARDIOGRAM IS DISCONNECTED BEFORE DISCHARGING THE DEFIBRILLATOR. ALSO DISCONNECT OTHER ELECTRICAL APPARATUS. Leave the bedside monitor connected. The graphic recorder at the central station need not be disconnected. After the shock is delivered, check the ECG or monitor to assess the type of rhythm present.

Summary, Step 1
a. Defibrillate.

Step 2. If the patient is still fibrillating, inject 0.5 ml. of 1:1,000 or 5 ml. of 1:10,000 aqueous Adrenalin IV or intracardiac. Give this 1 or 2 minutes to circulate by means of external cardiac massage. This is intended to increase the height and strength of the fibrillatory waves and thus increase the chance for defibrillation. After allowing time for circulation, use the defibrillator again, as outlined in Step 1.

Summary, Step 2
a. Adrenalin.
b. Defibrillate.

Step 3. If fibrillation is still present, repeat the previous dose of Adrenalin and, in addition, give 5–10 ml. of 10% calcium chloride or calcium gluconate IV. Allow to circulate, then again attempt defibrillation.

Summary, Step 3
a. Adrenalin.
b. Calcium gluconate.
c. Defibrillate.

Step 4. If the patient is still fibrillating, repeat the Adrenalin and calcium chloride again and, in addition, give 50–100 mg. lidocaine or 200 mg. of Pronestyl. Then give 1 or 2 shocks in succession.

Summary, Step 4
a. Adrenalin.
b. Calcium gluconate.
c. Lidocaine or Pronestyl.
d. 1 or 2 shocks in succession.

Step 5. If at any time, the patient converts to a rhythm other than ventricular fibrillation, give 50–100 mg.

lidocaine or 200 mg. Pronestyl IV. Even if the patient then reverts to ventricular fibrillation or ventricular tachycardia, the lidocaine or Pronestyl injection should be completed, then defibrillation again attempted, starting again with Step 1.

TYPES OF ARREST THAT CANNOT BE DEFIBRILLATED

1. Ventricular standstill (asystole).
2. Slow idioventricular rhythm.
3. Extreme sinus bradycardia.
4. Profound cardiovascular collapse.

The prognosis for the rhythms listed above is worse than that for ventricular fibrillation. *These rhythms will not respond to the defibrillator,* and all therapy is aimed at improving the strength and rate of contraction.

THERAPY

1. Isoproterenol (Isuprel) is the drug of choice. Begin with 0.1 or 0.2 mg. IV, and if a satisfactory increase in rate is noted, start 500 ml. of 5% D/W with 1 mg. Isuprel as a drip at the rate of infusion needed to maintain cardiac rate.
2. If Isuprel alone does not satisfactorily increase the rate, administer 2 mg. Isuprel in 500 ml. of 5% D/W and in addition give Adrenalin, 0.5 ml. of 1:1,000 or 5 ml. of 1:10,000 IV. This can be repeated as needed.
3. Aramine, if it is being infused along with bicarbonate, may be increased to 200 mg./1,000 ml. if this is necessary to raise or to maintain the blood pressure.
4. If these measures do not result in any increase in rate or pressure, 5–10 ml. of 10% calcium chloride or calcium gluconate may be injected slowly, IV, in an attempt to increase myocardial tone.
5. Atropine, 0.4–1 mg. IV, is the drug of choice for extreme sinus bradycardia.
6. The external pacemaker is unsatisfactory, in that it does not pace reliably and causes great patient discomfort. *An intravenous pacemaker is the method of choice when the patient becomes stabilized.*

Procedures for Physicians and Nurses

Central Venous Pressure (CVP)

USES FOR CENTRAL VENOUS PRESSURE

1. Detection of impending congestive heart failure, cardiac overload and development of pulmonary edema.
2. A guide to the rate of fluid volume administration.
3. A route for drug administration.
4. Access for taking blood samples or phlebotomy.
5. Intra-atrial ECG—for better detection of P-waves (via wire and saline bridge).

RANGES OF CENTRAL VENOUS PRESSURE

Normal ranges are as follows:
1. 2–10 cm. water—normal.
2. 10–15 cm. water—borderline.
3. Above 15 cm. water indicates that the heart is unable to accept the volume of blood that is returned from the circulation, for whatever reason.
4. N.B.: *Relative* readings are more important than one reading. Increases and decreases are significant.

TECHNIQUE

1. A polyethylene radiopaque catheter 33–36 in. long with an adequate hub at the outside end is inserted. (Commercially prepared units are available.)
   a. Insertion is usually via percutaneous needle; surgical cutdown may be used.
2. The catheter is positioned transvenously into the superior vena cava or the right atrium.
   a. Determine that it is properly positioned by measurement of the CVP and by determining that changes in CVP occur with respiration and the Valsalva maneuver.
3. The catheter is attached to a 3-way stopcock and manometer, and the IV tubing (from fluids bottle) is attached to the stopcock.
4. The height of the 3-way stopcock (zero on the manometer) is adjusted to the midaxillary line with the patient in the supine position.
   a. Accuracy of the pressure reading depends on the position of the patient relative to the level of the stopcock (zero on the manometer).
5. *Note:* The relative changes in CVP as measured by one individual with the patient in a standard position and correlated with clinical findings is of primary importance.
6. Numerous commercial CVP catheters, manometers and connection methods are available today. For the correct technique required to insert and attach a specific type of commercial catheter–manometer set-up, consult the manufacturer's literature accompanying the items.
7. The *hazards* of long-line CVP catheters in place are essentially those of short IV catheters at the puncture site, namely, phlebitis, thrombosis, embolism and cannula sepsis; those of the mechanical problems associated with transvenous electrode catheters; and the formation of a clot at the end of the CVP catheter opening.

Installation of Transvenous Electrode Catheter and External Pacemaker

PURPOSE

To install cardiac catheter into right ventricle by way of the jugular (or other) vein, through superior vena cava into right atrium, through tricuspid valve into right ventricle—to provide external electrical stimulus to ventricles.

EQUIPMENT

1. IV with Isuprel.
   a. Physician will order amount.
2. Gooseneck lamp.
3. Crash cart.
4. Pacemaker with battery.
5. Cardiac catheter and set of alligator clips (sterile).
6. Cardiac catheter pack.
   a. If scheduled, Surgery will put up own pack.
   b. If emergency, pack will come from Central Supply.
7. Dressing cart.
8. Microdrip Venopak.
9. Surgical Venopak.
10. Adhesive tape, 1″ and 2″.
11. Elastoplast, 2″ roll.

PROCEDURE

1. This is usually an emergency procedure.
   a. Observe the patient carefully for vital signs, congestive failure, etc., while preparing for procedure.
   b. Patient could require Code Blue before procedure starts.
2. The procedure may be done in X-ray or can be done in the unit.
3. If patient is in ccu, notify:
   a. Surgery for scrub nurse.
   b. Anesthesia.
   c. ECG.
   d. Central Service.
   e. Nursing Office.
   f. X-ray for portable equipment and plenty of chest films.
4. Operative permit should be properly signed and witnessed.
5. Preoperative sedation is given as ordered.
6. Place patient on lead I or II and connect to monitor.

a. Patient may already be on monitor.
7. Check battery in pacemaker for date.
   a. Life of battery is 6 months on the shelf. If battery has been used more than 4 hours intermittently or 3 days continuously, it is to be discarded and a new battery inserted with current date at time of insertion. Life of battery when in use is 500 hours or 21 days.
   b. Turn pacemaker on to see if it is working properly.
      1) Demand pacemaker has a bouncing red needle when turned on.
      2) Constant pacemaker has a flashing light when turned on.
8. If IV is not going, start 1,000 ml. of 5% D/W with B-D needle in right arm with surgical Venopak.
   a. Have Isuprel drip with microdrip Venopak piggy-backed at needle, ready to use if needed.
9. May have to prep the patient.
   a. Use disposable prep tray if Surgery does not bring one.
      1) Use prep that doctor orders.
10. Place gooseneck lamp in correct position.
    a. Turn bedside light on.
11. Physician will order chest film whenever necessary.
    a. Assist x-ray technician in placing and removing film.
12. When doctor is ready to check catheter placement, he will hand you the 2 tips of the alligator clips to attach to the pacemaker box. Be sure to attach the positive tip to the positive connector and the negative tip to the negative connector.
13. Observe scope and see if R-wave is preceded by a pacer "blip."
    a. Run frequent tracings.
14. When properly in place, tape with adhesive tape or Elastoplast.
15. Attach catheter to proper inlet in pacemaker.
16. Place ABD dressing between patient's chest and the pacemaker.
17. Secure pacemaker to chest with harness provided.
18. Check apical pulse for full minute and compare with rate the pacemaker is set on.
19. When the procedure is over, follow routine procedure for taking care of patient in ccu.
    a. IV may now be changed to Xylocaine or Pronestyl drip attached piggy-back to surgical Venopak tubing.
    b. Leave both Isuprel and Xylocaine attached temporarily for ready availability.

CCU Nursing Routines

Orders for Care of Acute Myocardial Infarction Patient

1. Start O₂ by suitable route, including IPPB and Ambu, as needed.

2. Call Anesthesia for endotracheal intubation in event of cardiac arrest.
3. Initiate cardiac massage, when needed, and respiratory assistance by appropriate method.

TABLE 10.—Guide to Dilutions and Dosages for Parenteral Medications
(Note: Use Microdrip for Infusion = 60 Gtts./Ml.)

Drug (Generic/Trade)	Package	Single Dose	Dilution	Dilution Concentration	Infusion Rate	Comments
Lidocaine (Xylocaine)	1% = 0.5 Gm./50 ml. 2% = 1.0 Gm./50 ml.	25-100 mg. IV bolus	0.5 Gm./250 ml. } 1 Gm./500 ml. } 0.2%	2 mg./ml.	1-5 mg./min. Titrate	Usual therapy; bolus followed by infusion
			2.5 Gm./500 ml. } 5 Gm./1000 ml. } 0.5%	5 mg./ml.		
Procainamide (Pronestyl)	1.0 Gm./10 ml. (100 mg./ml.)	500-750 mg. IM 50-200 mg. IV	1 Gm./50 ml. 1 Gm./250 ml.	20 mg./ml. 4 mg./ml.	25-50 mg./min. Maximum 250-500 mg./hr. Titrate 40 mg./min.	Observe for hypotension with IV administration
Quinidine Gluconate	0.8 Gm./10 ml. (80 mg./ml.)		0.8 Gm./50 ml. 0.8 Gm./250 ml.	16 mg./ml. 3.2 mg./ml.		Not recommended IV; monitor ECG and blood pressure
Diphenylhydantoin (Dilantin)	250 mg./5 ml.	125-250 mg. IV	250 mg./10 ml. 250 mg./25 ml.	25 mg./ml. 10 mg./ml.	1 mg./kg./min. (250 mg./3-5 min.)	Slow injection mandatory
Propranolol (Inderal)	1 mg./1 ml.	1-3 mg.			0.5-1 mg./min.	Slow injection mandatory
Atropine sulfate	8 mg./20 ml. (0.4 mg./ml.)	0.3-2 mg. IV or 0.3 mg. increments to total of 2 mg.	2 mg./50 ml.	0.04 mg./ml.	0.05-0.1 mg./kg./5 min. 0.04 mg./min. (1 ml./min.) (0.4 mg./10 min.) Titrate	
Edrophonium (Tensilon)	10 mg./ml. 100 mg./10 ml.	10 mg. IV bolus				Chiefly diagnostic agent
Digitalis	See Table 5.					
Isoproterenol (Isuprel)	1 mg./5 ml.		1-2 mg./500 ml. (for bradyarrhythmia)	2-4 µg./ml.	5 µg. (2.5-1.25 ml.)/min. Then titrate	Beta sympathomimetic agent; may be more dilute or concentrated, depending on patient fluid needs.
			1 mg./500 ml. (for cardiogenic shock)	2 µg./ml.	Titrate	For cardiogenic shock
Norepinephrine (Levophed)	4 mg. base/4 ml.		4-16 mg. base/1,000 ml.	4-16 µg./ml.	Start-2-4 µg./min. Then titrate	Norepinephrine-liberating drug
Metaraminol (Aramine)	10 mg./1 ml. 100 mg./10 ml.	2-10 mg. IM	50 mg./500 ml. 100 mg./1,000 ml.	0.1 mg./ml.	Titrate	
Epinephrine (Adrenalin)	1 ml. (1:1,000) 30 ml. (1:1,000)	5-10 cc. of 1:10,000 IV	1 ml. of 1:1,000 (1 mg.) in 500 ml.	2 µg./ml.	1-2 ml./min.	For resuscitation
Potassium chloride –KCL	40 mEq./20 ml.		40 mEq./500 ml.		40 mEq./hr. maximum	For digitalis toxicity; give at even infusion rate
Sodium bicarbonate –NaHCO₃	44 mEq./50 ml. 500 ml. of 5% solution (5 Gm./100 ml.)	44 mEq. (50 ml.) (3.36 Gm.) IV			Give every 8-10 min. Rate of 75 ml. every 5 min. (15 ml./min.)	For acidosis; used for cardiopulmonary resuscitation
Molar sodium lactate	40 mEq./40 ml.	10-80 ml. IV	Molar or half-molar		4-10 ml./min.	For acidosis
Calcium gluconate	1 Gm./10 ml. (10%)	1 gm. (10 ml. of 10%) IV or intracardiac				For cardiopulmonary resuscitation

4. Start IV, preferably via plastic needle.
5. ECG (direct writer) is to be taken whenever needed to ascertain arrhythmia. Inform attending physician of development of any arrhythmia.
6. Start 500 ml. sodium bicarbonate in event of cardiac arrest.
7. Use defibrillator in ventricular fibrillation, if physician is not available after suitable documentation, and if case justifies this procedure of resuscitation.
8. Use defibrillator in ventricular tachycardia, if sustained, and if not responding to any of the following:
   a. Xylocaine, 25–50 mg. as IV bolus, repeated as indicated, or
   b. IV Pronestyl, 1,000 mg./1,000 ml., or
   c. Xylocaine, 1–2 mg./minute in IV.
   d. Suitable documentation of ventricular tachycardia will be necessary, and the patient must show evidence of collapse.
9. Atropine, 0.3–1.2 mg. IV is given by nurse in the event sinus bradycardia develops or in patient presenting with this rhythm.
10. IV Pronestyl or Xylocaine, as outlined above, is given by nurse in the event VPCs occur (a) early (on top of T-wave), (b) in salvos, (c) multiple foci, or (d) sustained and more than 5/minute.
11. Have Isuprel (1 mg. ampules) ready with microdrip for IV use, in the event of increasing 2d- or 3d-degree heart block. Do not administer without physician's instructions.
12. Have transvenous catheter and battery pacemaker ready for insertion in patient with complete heart block. Alert physician as to changes in condition.
13. Once right ventricular catheter is in place and on standby, nurse may put pacemaker on battery-powered operation immediately in the event of asystole or an Adams-Stokes episode.

In a Community Hospital

1. Nursing Notebook Standard Orders: to be considered a part of the routine to the following orders where they apply.
2. Vital signs: as per CCU Vital Signs routing in Nursing Notebook.
3. Monitoring: as per CCU Monitoring Procedure routine in Nursing Notebook.
4. Initiate Code Blue procedure if cardiac arrest occurs, as described in Nursing Notebook.
5. Notify physician of development of any arrhythmias, as per Nursing Notebook.
6. Notify physician of respiratory distress, increasing cough or rattling respiration.
7. O₂ by nasal cannula at 5 L./minute unless otherwise specified.
8. Absolute bedrest.
9. Side rails up at all times.
10. 900 calorie liquid diet.
11. No hot or cold liquids.
12. No coffee or tea—may have Sanka.
13. 24-hour intake and output.
14. Insert B-D needle—with obturator—or fluids as ordered by physician.
15. Other orders as per attending physician.

Coronary Care Patient Routine

Purposes

1. To aid in the return of the coronary patient to normal as quickly as possible.
2. To use direct and mechanical observation and professional judgment to protect patient against further cardiac damage if diagnosis of myocardial infarction is made.
3. To observe patient closely to help diagnose myocardial infarction.

Procedure

1. Absolute bedrest—no reading, radio or TV unless ordered.
2. Complete bedbath.
   a. Daily bath as patient's condition warrants.
      1) May need rest more than bath.
3. Feed patient.
   a. May be fed by relative if condition warrants.
4. No hot or ice-cold liquids.
5. No coffee or tea.
   a. Sanka only, unless otherwise ordered by physician.
6. Oxygen whenever necessary.
   a. No rectal temperature is taken without physician's order. Take oral temperature with oxygen going.
7. Monitor all patients.
   a. Limb or chest leads; lead II most commonly used.
   b. Electrode plates, if used, to be cleaned once each shift and reapplied.
      1) Clean with cleanser, Rescue pad and toothbrush.
   c. Semi-floating adhesive electrodes may be used.
8. Full lead ECG whenever condition warrants.
9. Oral hygiene every 4 hours if needed.
10. Turn every 2 hours.
11. Side rails up at all times.
12. Insert B-D needle on all coronary patients and add IV fluids on physician's orders.
13. Lifeguard pulse alarms to be set 20 points below pulse rate and also 20 points above.
14. Automatic printers to be on remote at all times.
    a. Paper is inexpensive when it comes to recording an arrhythmia that may develop in a patient.
15. If oral and nasal suction is used, the bottle suction unit, tubing, Y-connector, nasal catheter and IV bottle containing aqueous Zephiran 1:750 is to be changed daily by the 11–7 shift and an all new set-up reapplied.

a. The nurse on 11-7 will rinse bottles and leave for personnel on the 7-3 shift to wash and send to Central Supply for sterilizing.

b. Suction bottles are to be emptied and rinsed out on the 7-3 and 3-11 shifts.

16. The nurse may defibrillate when condition warrants and follow CCU Nursing Orders for care of acute myocardial infarction, when signed by the physician for that individual patient.

17. Accurate 24-hour intake and output with or without doctor's orders.

a. For intake of oral fluids, use measured paper cup only.

b. Record when cup is empty and not after each sip.

18. Comatose patient receives eye care once each shift.

a. Order eye tray.

19. If patient gets phlebitis from plastic needle, may put warm wet packs to area.

CCU Vital Signs Routine

PURPOSE

1. Adequate observation of patient's vital signs to gather information necessary for treatment and diagnosis and still provide adequate rest for recovery.

2. Because each patient's condition differs, individual evaluation is necessary to determine how often vital signs must be ascertained to be of value.

Procedure

1. Apical pulse (AP) is routinely taken. If unable to obtain AP (chest congestion), notation is made on vital signs sheet as to pulse location.

a. RP — radial pulse.

b. CP — carotid pulse.

c. FP — femoral pulse.

d. PP — pedal pulse.

2. BP–AP–R

15 minutes × 4 necessary. Then

20 minutes × 1; value to this patient.

60 minutes × 1; value to this patient.

2 hours × 2; value to this patient.

Then every 4 hours, with constant alertness that the patient's need may change. Above is the minimum frequency. Take additional readings as indicated.

3. V/S (vital signs) are taken every 15 minutes on patient receiving vasopressor medication until pressure is stabilized; then V/S may be taken every 30 minutes with the realization that patient's condition needs constant evaluation.

4. T.P.R. (temperature, pulse, respiration) are taken every 4 hours and recorded on chart as well as on special graphic sheet. No rectal temperatures are taken on cardiac patients without physician's orders.

a. Axillary temperatures are not generally acceptable; oral may be taken with O_2 catheter or cannula in place.

Procedure for Rotating Tourniquets

PURPOSE

1. To relieve acute pulmonary edema.

2. To obstruct venous blood return to the heart.

EQUIPMENT

1. 3 rubber tourniquets or blood pressure cuffs.

2. Sedation as prescribed by physician.

PROCEDURE

1. Place tourniquets on 3 extremities at a time.

a. Arm tourniquet should be placed approximately 4 in. below shoulder.

b. Thigh tourniquet should be placed approximately 6 in. below groin. (Volume of blood held out by tourniquet: 1 leg equals 2 arms.)

c. Maintain tourniquet pressure greater than venous pressure, but less than arterial.

2. Rotate every 15 minutes or as ordered by physician.

a. Color must return to extremity each time tourniquet is off the limb.

1) If color does not return, notify physician at once.

3. Record on special graphic sheet at bedside the time and order of rotation.

a. E.g., 1:00 RA, 1:15 RL, 1:30 LL, 1:45 LA, 2:00 RA.

4. Continue until emergency is over or physician discontinues.

a. Take off one tourniquet at a time, every 5-15 minutes.

Chart for Bedside and Emergency Medication Charting

CONSTRUCTION OF CHART

1. A chart of this type should be constructed in *graphic form* so that divisions of time may be indicated for whatever time intervals are necessary for the specific patient.

2. A blood pressure graphic section may be so constructed that blood pressure readings may be entered on an individual basis (i.e., written into the graphic form rather than having fixed blood pressure readings printed on the chart form).

ITEMS TO CONSIDER

1. Date.

2. Time.

3. Hospital day.

4. Temperature.

5. Pulse.

6. Respirations.

7. Intake.

8. Urine output.

9. Other items specific for cardiac function, e.g.:
   a. Arrhythmia present?
   b. VPCs/minute.
   c. Central venous pressure.
10. Blood pressure graphic section.
11. Blood studies section may be desirable.
12. Medications and intravenous fluids.
    a. Used particularly for entering medications utilized in treating the complications of acute myocardial infarction.
    b. Intravenous fluids entered are those which contain medications used for complications of acute myocardial infarction.
13. *Comments.*
    a. Date and time on all entries.
    b. Initial or sign all entries.

Flow Chart for Cardiac Arrest

CONSTRUCTION OF FLOW CHART

By taking into account the drugs potentially administered and the procedures that might be undertaken on a patient with cardiac arrest in the CCU, a chart can be devised that is best fitted for the specific institution. An excellent example is available in the literature.[36]

ITEMS TO CONSIDER

Suggested therapeutic items are to be listed horizontally, with the time and the amount of therapeutic item listed vertically.
1. Time.
2. Blood pressure (mm./Hg).
3. Heart rate/minute.
4. Levarterenol.
5. Metaraminol.
6. Epinephrine.
7. Isoproterenol.
8. Calcium chloride or gluconate (10 ml. of 10% solution/vial).
9. Sodium bicarbonate.
10. Procainamide.
11. Lidocaine.
12. Digitalis.
13. Electrical cardioversion.
14. Others.
15. Comments.

RESPONSIBILITY AND METHODOLOGY FOR RECORDING INFORMATION

1. Responsibility for recording the information concerning a cardiac arrest and the ensuing cardiopulmonary resuscitation must be assumed by supervisory nursing personnel if at all possible. If this is not possible, other arrangements must be made specific to the situation of the individual CCU. Make the arrangements in advance.

2. Time entries should be made according to actual time from a clock with a second hand.
3. If the unit has an elapsed timer(s), the actual time should be correlated with the elapsed time early in the cardiopulmonary resuscitation.

Intake and Output (I and O) Information and Charting

FLUID BALANCE SHEET CONTENTS

Parenteral Intake (ml.)

1. Type of fluids (include added electrolytes).
2. Start time.
3. Finish time.
4. Amount received.
   a. By shift.
   b. 24-hour total.

Enteral Intake (ml.)

1. Tube.
2. Oral.
3. Record by shift and 24-hour total.

Output

1. Vomitus or suction.
2. Ostomy.
3. Urine.
   a. Catheter.
   b. Voided.
4. By shift and 24-hour total.
5. More frequently on work sheet if condition warrants.

Exact Makeup of the Form

There are many forms for Intake and Output (I and O) designed for individual hospitals which permit adequate and accurate recording of intake and output.

MEMOS CONCERNING INTAKE AND OUTPUT

Simple Method of Calculating IV Fluid, Rates and Amounts

1. Always break down your calculation to amounts in 1 hour; then you can easily figure 8-hour shift and 24-hour amounts.
2. The number of drops/minute × 4 = the number of milliliters (ml.)/ hour (e.g., 40 gtts./minute × 4 = 160 ml./hour).
3. The number of milliliters/hour ÷ 4 = the number of drops/minute (e.g., 200 ml. ÷ 4 = 50 gtts./minute).
4. 4 microdrops = 1 macrodrop (regular IV drop).
5. The number of microdrops/minute = the number of milliliters/hour (e.g., 50 microdrops/minute = 50 ml./hour).

Accurate Measurement of Every Milliliter Given to Patient

1. This can be done as frequently as necessary, depending on the patient's condition. Every 1, 2, 3, 4 or 8 hours.
2. Precalibrate the amount of solution to be given on your shift. Place a narrow strip of tape on the bottle along the calibrate. Use this to mark at the end of each shift, so the person on the next shift knows where to start figuring. Mark these tapes at 6:00 A.M., 2:00 P.M. and 10:00 P.M. Number bottles consecutively.
3. Make sure that all IV bottles used are accounted for at the close of your shift. Keep the used bottles until your totals are accounted for on the patient's chart.
4. Microdrop IV tubings should be used on all patients in Intensive Care unless there is a need to force IV fluids. On other floors either the macro or micro can be used.
5. Careful communication with persons on next shift regarding fluids given is essential.
6. Oral intake must be accounted for as accurately as IV fluids. This includes ice chips and water given with medications.
7. Any medication added to the IV should be accounted for as well as IV push medications. Remember to calculate the excess of each bottle unless you have spilled it out before starting the IV.

   Abbott bottle excess 1,000 ml.   30–40
                     500 ml.   30–40
                     250 ml.   30–40
                     150 ml.   30–40
8. Fluid used for lavage of nasogastric tubes, bladder, etc., must not be disregarded.

Accurate Measurement of Output from Patient

1. Urine should be measured each hour or more frequently on every patient with a labile cardiac condition. In other cardiac patients, accurate measurement of urine is requisite but may be done less frequently.
2. If the patient is unable to void on the hour, use of a Foley catheter may be indicated, and the physician should be consulted. Repeated straight catheterizations increase the possibility of bladder infection.
3. For convenience, outputs are measured on the hour. Prior to collection of the specimen, make sure the bladder is empty. Positioning may be necessary. All urine in tubing is drained into collection receptacle. Always check for plugs and kinks in the drainage system.

Insensible Loss

This includes moisture lost from the GI tract, the respiratory tract and the skin.

1. GI tract.
   a. Emesis.
   b. Stool amount, number and consistency.
   c. Gastrointestinal tubes, e.g., nasogastric, T-tube, gastrostomy.
2. Respiratory tract.
   a. Mouth breathing increases loss of moisture.
   b. Hyperventilation results in more fluid loss than does normal breathing.
   c. Record accurately the type of respirations.
   d. Less moisture is lost through this route if moist air is being inhaled.
3. Skin.
   a. Diaphoresis—extent and duration.
   b. Temperature. Febrile patient loses more moisture than the afebrile.
4. Miscellaneous (paracentesis, etc.).

Representative Contents of Fluid Containers

Ice tea glass	300 ml.
8 oz. water glass	240 ml.
6 oz. water glass	180 ml.
Juice glass	100 ml.
Coffee cup	125 ml.
Soup bowl	125 ml.

Intravenous (IV) Therapy

THE PRIMARY IV

Attach a primary IV to maintain an opening into the venous system for later urgent or emergency use should IV medications become necessary.

1. Primary IV fluids should contain no medication and should utilize microdrip tubing.
2. Secure the IV by a plastic cannula arrangement of some sort that will permit the patient to move his arm about and that will hold the IV more securely in place than would be the case if a needle were used. One of the following may be used:
   a. B-D Teflon catheter. Attach with fluids and IV tubing, or place an obturator in the Teflon needle for later rapid attachment of IV set-up.
   b. Intracath or other polyethylene catheter.
   c. Central venous pressure catheter set-up for CVP readings as well as fluids.
3. Use a long tubing from the fluids bottle to the patient, thus permitting greater mobility of fluids and apparatus.
4. Place large-bore tubing in the vein. The limiting factor to the speed of IV drip is in most instances the diameter of the IV catheter.
5. Before placing the primary IV cannula (catheter), prepare the skin with antiseptic technique if at all possible.

6. An antibiotic ointment applied to the site the tubing penetrates the skin has been noted to decrease the incidence of infection.

SECONDARY IV

1. Infusions should be attached at the site of needle acceptance (rubber plug or bulb) in the primary IV tubing which is nearest the patient.
2. This leaves the shortest possible column of fluid containing the nonmedication primary fluids or the medication-containing secondary fluids, when making a change from one source of fluids to another.
3. Secondary units should probably use the microdrip tubing (60 gtts./ml.).
4. More than one secondary unit may be attached to the tube needle acceptance site nearest the patient.
5. Each secondary unit should be regulated by the regulation mechanism on the tubing that leads from that particular unit.

LABEL ALL BOTTLES CONTAINING MEDICATION

1. Label as to type of medication, quantity of medication and the date mixed. The time of placement of the fluids bottle is also desirable.
2. The bottles should be numbered sequentially for each patient during his stay in the coronary care unit.

IV MEDICATION

1. IV medication (not mixed in the bottle of fluids for IV infusion) should be given into the primary tubing at the site nearest the patient.
2. This applies for both bolus medication and slow IV medication.
3. Medication for slow IV use should be adequately diluted so as to help prevent rapid injection of a concentrated solution.
4. Individual injection speed depends on the medication and the circumstances.
5. Remove the same volume of fluid from the fluids bottle that will be added when medication is mixed into a bottle for use as IV infusion.
   a. Individual coronary care units may permit 10 ml. or so to be added without removing a like amount.
   b. Some units may desire that fluids be removed from the bottle to permit *exact* dilutions.

STARTING AND MAINTAINING IV

1. The maintenance of a venous catheter for a relatively long time, as is usually done in the CCU, presents the possible hazards of phlebitis, thrombosis, embolism and cannula sepsis. In studies done after proper preparation of the skin and proper maintenance of the skin puncture site, 5% or less of the catheters cultured have shown bacteria grown from their tips. Those that have given positive results have shown staphylococcus.[267,268] Therefore it is extremely important that the skin site be properly prepared to keep complications to a minimum.
2. The following is a suggested routine for starting and maintaining the IV catheter.
   a. Shave the skin, if necessary.
   b. Prepare with isopropyl alcohol (99% isopropanol).
   c. Blot dry with sterile gauze.
   d. Paint with povidone-iodine (Betadine) and allow to dry before inserting catheter.
   e. Inspect catheter site at least daily.
   f. May desire topical antibiotic (e.g., bacitracin) applied at catheter site.
   g. If local evidence of phlebitis or cellulitis appears, remove the catheter from this site and treat as indicated.
   h. A larger bore vein is less likely to be irritated by the catheter and medications passing through it than is a small-bore vein.
3. If the hospital staff can properly maintain them, scalp vein needles may cause less irritation.

The Metric System of Measurements

ADVANTAGES

The metric system[238] permits the correlation, interchange and consistent interaction of all types of measurements without conversion to a different system or systems of units. It permits conversion into all quantities of weight and volume within the same system, and it may be used internationally for all measurements.

Weight/volume relationships may be utilized with easy interchange and calculation of various concentrations and dilutions. Therefore, dosages should be expressed in metric units rather than in any other system of weights and measurements. The metric system also adapts well to the decimal system.

UNITS OF MEASUREMENT

1. *Weight*
   Kilogram (kg.) = 1,000 Gm. (approx. 2.2 lb.)
   Gram (Gm.) = 1,000 mg. = 1/1,000 kg.
   Milligram (mg.) = 1,000 μg. = 1/1,000 Gm.
   Microgram (μg.) = 1/1,000 mg.
   Milliequivalent (mEq.) = equivalent weight expressed in milligrams.
2. *Volume*
   Liter (L.) 1,000 ml. (approx. 1 qt.)
   Milliliter (ml.) = 1/1,000 L. = 1 cc. = 1 cubic centimeter of liquid.
3. *Distance*
   Centimeter (cm.) = 10 mm. (approx. 2.4 cm. = 1 in.)
   Millimeter (mm.) = 0.1 cm.
4. *Other related measurements*
   1 ounce (oz.) = 30 cc.
   1/2 ounce = 15 cc. = 1 tablespoon
   1 teaspoon = approx. 5 cc.
   1 grain (gr.) = 64 mg.
   1/150 gr. = 0.4 mg.

Glossary
(DEFINITIONS AND VOCABULARY)

ACTION POTENTIAL: The electrical charge (change of electrical potential) as it is propagated along a conduction system.

ACCU: Acute coronary care unit; same as CCU and ICCU.

ACH: Acetylcholine.

ADENOSINE: A nucleotide, adenine-D-ribose, derived from the nucleic acid adenine.

ADP: Adenosine diphosphate. The nucleotide adenosine plus diphosphate.

ADRENERGIC: Same as Sympathetic. Derived from the fact that adrenalin was the first chemical found to be a final chemical mediator of sympathetic nerve impulses.

AEROBIC: In the presence of oxygen.

AFFERENT: The fibers going *to* the CNS, or the impulse flowing *toward* the CNS.

ALEVEOLI: The air cells of the lungs.

ALVEOLUS: An air sac (singular form) of the lungs formed by terminal dilatations of the bronchioles.

AMI: Acute myocardial infarction.

AMP: Adenosine monophosphate. The nucleotide adenosine plus monophosphate.

ANAEROBIC: In the absence of free oxygen.

ANALOGS: Chemicals (medications) similar in function or structure.

ANASARCA: An accumulation of fluid in all the tissues of the body; general edema and ascites.

ANOXIA: Without oxygen.

ANTI-: Against

APC: Atrial premature contraction (PAC).

APNEA: No breathing.

ARRHYTHMIA: Lack of rhythm.

ARTERIOLE: A small artery, especially one just proximal to a capillary.

ATARAXIC: Calming; tranquilizing.

ATP: Adenosine triphosphate: A nucleotide triphosphate compound occurring in all cells but particularly muscle tissue: represents the energy reserve of the muscle. The nucleotide adenosine plus triphosphate.

AUSCULTATION: The act of listening for sounds within the body.

AUTO-: Self.

AUTONOMIC NERVOUS SYSTEM: The so-called involuntary nervous system which controls the automatic functions of the body.

AV: Atrioventricular.

BI-: Two.

BIO-: Life.

BOLUS(ES): Mass(es) of medication given at one time.

BRADY-: Slow.

CAPACITANCE: Capacity of the microcirculation and its ability to change.

CAPILLARIES: The minute vessels which connect the arterioles and the venules, forming a network in nearly all parts of the body.

CAPILLARY LOOP: The term applied to the network of blood vessels, including arterioles, capillaries and venules

CARDI-: Heart.

CARDIAC ARRHYTHMIA: A disturbance in the rhythm of either the atria or ventricles (or both) of the heart.

CARDIAC TAMPONADE: Acute compression of the heart due to effusion of fluid into the pericardial sac.

CATALYSIS: Change in velocity of a reacton produced by presence of a substance which does not form part of the final product (i.e., the presence of a catalyst).

CATALYZE: To cause catalysis; to act as a catalyzer.

Cc: Cubic centimeter (ml.).

CCU: Coronary care unit; same as ACCU and ICCU.

CEPHALO-: Head.

CHELATING: Chemically binding.

CHF: Congestive heart failure.

CHOLINERGIC: Same as Parasympathetic. Derived from the fact that acetylcholine was found to be the final chemical mediator of the parasympathetic nerve impulse.

CHRONO-: Time.

141

CHRONOTROPIC EFFECT: To accelerate heart rate.

CNS: Central nervous system (the brain and spinal cord).

COLLATERAL CIRCULATION: That circulation which is carried on through secondary channels after stoppage of the principal channel.

COMPETITIVE INHIBITION: Arrest, restraint or change of a process by utilization of a closely similar compound to alter the effects of an essential metabolite.

CONDUCTIVITY: The capacity to conduct an electric current.

CONTRA-: Against.

CONTRACT: To draw together; to shorten

CONTRACTILE: Having the power or tendency to contract in response to a suitable stimulus.

CONTRACTILITY: Capacity for becoming short in response to a suitable stimulus.

CONTRAINDICATIONS: Indications against use.

CORONARY ANGIOGRAPHY: Radiopaque dye studies of the coronary arteries.

CUMULATIVE EFFECTS: The effects of accumulation of a drug in the body.

CUTANEOUS: Pertaining to the skin.

CVP: Central venous pressure.

CYANO-: Blue.

CYTO-: Cell.

DC: Direct current.

DEPOLARIZATION: Electrical activation.

DI-: Two.

DISCHARGE: Electrical discharge.

DISTAL: Farthest from the center, origin or head; opposed to proximal.

DYS-: Painful, bad, disordered.

DYSPNEA: Difficult breathing.

ECG (EKG): Electrocardiogram.

ECTO-: Outside.

ECTOPIC: Out of the normal place.

ECTOPIC FOCUS: A focus of origin of cardiac impulse located outside the normal place.

EDEMA: Presence of abnormally large amounts of fluid in the intracellular tissue spaces of the body.

EEG: Electroencephalogram.

EFFECTOR ORGAN: See End-organ.

EFFERENT: The fibers leading *from* the CNS, or the nerve impulse flowing *away from* the CNS.

EFFUSION: The escape of fluid into a part or tissue.

E.G.: For example.

EMBOLUS: A clot or other plug brought by the blood current from a distant vessel and forced into a smaller one so as to obstruct the circulation.

EMBOLISM: The sudden blocking of an artery or vein by a clot or obstruction which has been brought to its place by the blood current.

-EMIA: Blood.

EN-: In.

END-ORGAN (EFFECTOR ORGAN): Term usually used to indicate the organ system influenced by the impulses that travel down the neurons of the efferent pathways of the autonomic nervous system. (Also a nerve end-organ which serves to distribute impulses which activate muscle contraction and gland stimulation.)

ENDO-: Within.

ENDOGENOUS: Within the body.

ENZYME: An organic compound, frequently a protein, capable of accelerating (or catalyzing) a chemical reaction. The chemical reaction involves the substrate (compound) on which the enzyme acts and for which the enzyme is usually specific.

EPI-: On or upon.

EX-: Out.

EXOGENOUS: Outside the body.

FLUX: A flow, usually back and forth across a partition (as in transmembrane flux or flow across a membrane).

GLYCO-: Sweet, sugarlike.

GLYCOGENOLYSIS: The splitting up of glycogen in the body tissues.

-gram: Mark, writing.

-graphy: To write; to record.

HALF-LIFE: The time required for half of the drug to disappear from the bloodstream.

HEM- (HEMA-, HEMO-): Blood.

HEMOPERICARDIUM: Blood in the pericardial sac surrounding the heart.

HYDROLYSIS: Chemical breakdown of a molecule with the incorporation and splitting of water; the 2 resulting products divide the water; hydroxyl group to one resultant molecule and hydrogen atom to the other resultant molecule.

HYPER-: Over.

HYPO-: Under.

HYPOCAPNIA: Deficiency of carbon dioxide in the blood.

HYPOKALEMIA: Low serum potassium content.

HYPOTHESIS: A supposition assumed as a basis of reasoning.

HYPOVOLEMIA: Low intravascular fluid volume.

HYPOXEMIA: Same as Hypoxia in usual clinical usage.

HYPOXIA: Below normal levels of oxygen.

-IASIS: Resulting from.

-IATRIC: Pertaining to medicine.

IC: Intracardiac.

ICCU: Intensive coronary care unit.

I.E.: In other words; that is.

IM: Intramuscular.

INFARCT: An area of coagulation necrosis in a tissue due to lack of blood supply, resulting from obstruction of circulation to the area.

INFARCTION: The formation of an infarct.

INHIBIT: Prevent or stop.

INHIBITION: Arrest or restraint of a process.

INTER-: Between.

INTERSTITIAL: Pertaining to the interspaces of a tissue; the spaces between cells and connective fibers.

INTRA-: Within.

INTRINSIC: Situated entirely within itself.

INOTROPIC EFFECT: To increase the strength of myocardial contractility.

ION: An atom or group of atoms having a charge of positive or negative electricity.

IONIC: Pertaining to ion or ions.

ISCHEMIA: Local and temporary deficiency of blood, chiefly due to the constriction of a blood vessel.

ISO-: Equal.

IV: Intravenous.

KINETICS: The dynamics of equilibrium.

KG: Kilogram.

LIGATION: The application of a ligature.

LIGATURE: A thread or wire for tying a vessel or strangulating a part.

-LYSIS: Destruction.

MACRO-: Large.

MEDIATION: The action of serving as an intermediary.

METABOLISM: (a) tissue change; (b) the biochemical transformation by which energy is made available for uses of the organism.

METABOLITE: A biochemical which is involved in the process of metabolism.

μG: Microgram.

MG: Milligram.

MI: Myocardial infarction.

MICRO-: Small.

ML.: Milliliter.

MOLECULAR: Of, pertaining to or composed of molecules.

MOLECULE: A chemical combination of 2 or more atoms which form a specific chemical substance.

MONITOR: To observe on a continuous basis.

MONO-: One.

MORBIDITY: Illness.

MULTI-: Many.

-MYO-: Muscle.

MYOCARDIUM (Myo—muscle + Cardium—heart): The muscular substance of the heart; the heart muscle.

N.B.: Note well.

NECROSIS: Death of a cell or group of cells which is in contact with living tissue.

NERVE BLOCK: The blocking of the nerve impulse at some point along its pathway.

NERVE FIBER: A group of neurons forming a threadlike structure.

NEUROHORMONE: A chemical which transmits the nerve impulse.

NEUROHUMORAL: Same as Neurohormone.

NEUROHUMORAL SITE: The site at which the neurohormone (norepinephrine; acetylcholine) chemically transmits the nerve impulse (the ganglionic synapse and effector organ).

NEURON: A single nerve cell, consisting of body and axon.

NEUROTRANSMITTER: Same as Neurohormone.

NOREPINEPHRINE (LEVARTERENOL): The chemically active catecholamine neurotransmitter which is active at the peripheral sympathetic receptor site.

NPC: Nodal premature contraction (PNC).

OCCLUSION: The act of closure or state of being closed.

-OID: Form, like.

OLIGURIA: Reduced output of urine.

-OLOGY: Study of.

ORTHOPNEA: Inability to breathe except in an upright position.

OXIDIZE: To combine or cause to combine with oxygen. Increased positive charges on an atom, or loss of negative charges.

PAC: Premature atrial contraction (APC).

PARA-: Beside.

PARASYMPATHETIC NERVOUS SYSTEM: A division of the autonomic nervous system. The nerve impulses are chemically mediated by acetylcholine.

PARASYMPATHOLYTIC (Lytic—to lyse or destroy): Destroying (blocking) the effects of parasympathetic nervous system stimulation.

PARASYMPATHOMIMETIC (Mimetic—to imitate): Imitating the effects of parasympathetic nervous system stimulation.

PARAVERTEBRAL GANGLIONIC CHAIN: The chain of ganglia located on each side of the spinal column from the cervical to the sacral area, being divided into cervical, thoracic, lumbar and sacral portions, and being the site of synapse of the pre- with the postganglionic neurons of the sympathetic nervous system.

PARENTERAL: Inside the body, by IV, IM or subcutaneous injection.

PATHO-: Disease.

PATHOGENESIS: The process of development of morbid conditions of disease.

PATHOLOGIC PHYSIOLOGY: The study of disordered function or of function in diseased tissue.

PERCEIVE: To receive an impression through the senses.

PERCEPTION: The process or result of perceiving.

PERFUSION: The act of pouring over or through; the flow of blood through tissue.

PERI-: Around.

PERICARDIOCENTESIS: The surgical puncture of the pericardium for the purpose of aspirating pericardial effusions.

PERIHILAR: Around the hilum of the lungs.

PERMEABLE: Not impassable; pervious; that which may be traversed.

PHARMACOPHYSIOLOGY: The physiologic alterations caused by a pharmacologic agent (drug effect).

PHLEBOTOMY: Removal of blood through a vein.

PHOSPHORYLATION: Chemical addition of a phosphoric acid radical to another molecule.

PHOSPHOROLYSIS: A reversible combination and separation chemical reaction involving the phosphoric acid radical.

PLEXUS: A network or tangle of nerve fibers.

PNEUMO-: Lung.

PNC: Premature nodal contraction (NPC).

PND: Paroxysmal nocturnal dyspnea; dyspnea of sudden onset, occurring at night or in the recumbent position.

POSTGANGLIONIC: The neuron fibers originating in the paravertebral ganglionic chain in the sympathetic and in the peripheral plexus in the parasympathetic system and ending at the receptor site of the end-organ in both divisions of the autonomic nervous system.

POWER FAILURE: Same as Pump failure.

PRECURSOR: Forerunner of.

PREGANGLIONIC: The neuron fibers originating in the CNS and ending in the paravertebral ganglionic chain in the sympathetic division and in the peripheral organ plexus in the parasympathetic division.

PROGNOSIS: The prospect as to recovery from a disease.

PROTO-: First.

PROTOTYPE: The original type or form after which others are developed; an example of a class of drugs.

PROXIMAL: Nearest to the center, origin or head; opposed to distal.

PULMONARY CIRCULATION: The circulation of the blood through the lungs for the purpose of oxygenation. Also called the lesser circulation.

PULMONARY EDEMA: An effusion of serous fluid into the air sacs and interstitial tissue of the lungs.

PUMP FAILURE: Failure of the heart to function effectively as a pump.

PVC: Premature ventricular contraction (VPC).

RADIOGRAPHY: The making of a record or photograph by means of radioactivity; i.e., x-ray.

RECEPTOR SITE: A site (or sites) on a given end organ that receives only nerve impulses chemically mediated to that particular type of site. These receptor sites are chemically activated and chemically blocked in a selective manner.

REFRACTORY PERIOD, ABSOLUTE (ABSOLUTE REFRACTORY PERIOD): The period of time, following depolarization, when the conduction system will not respond to *any* form of stimulus. Repolarization is occurring during this period.

REFRACTORY PERIOD, EFFECTIVE (EFFECTIVE REFRACTORY PERIOD): The period of time, following depolarization, during which the conduction system will not carry a *propagated* impulse, though a stimulus may cause other active responses in the tissue.

REFRACTORY PERIOD, RELATIVE (RELATIVE REFRACTORY PERIOD): A period of time, *following* the absolute refractory period, during which the conduction system will respond, but *only* to a stimulus which is much stronger than normal. During this time conduction is also slower than normal.

RETRO-: Back, behind.

RETROGRADE: Backward.

SA: Sinoatrial.

-SCOPE: To view.

SOPORIFIC: Sleep-producing.

-STRIA-: Line or streak.

SUB-: Under, near, almost.

SUBSTRATE: The term applied to the substance upon which an enzyme acts.

SUPER-: Over.

SUPERFICIAL: Pertaining to or situated near the surface.

SUPRA-: Above.

SYMPATHETIC NERVOUS SYSTEM: A division of the autonomic nervous system. The nerve impulses are chemically mediated by norepinephrine.

SYMPATHOLYTIC (Lytic—to *lyse* or *destroy*): Destroying (blocking) the effects of sympathetic nervous system stimulation.

SYMPATHOMIMETIC (Mimetic—to *imitate*): Imitating the effects of sympathetic nervous system stimulation.

SYMPATHOMIMETIC AMINES: Chemical compounds which are either the same as the naturally occurring catecholamines of epinephrine and norepinephrine, or are closely related in chemical structure to these compounds and have the same effector organ results to a greater or lesser extent when introduced into the bloodstream. These amines are all of the same general class of drugs. The sympathomimetic amines are utilized in AMI predominantly in the treatment of cardiogenic shock.

SYNAPSE: The region of contact between processes of two adjacent neurons, forming the place where a nervous impulse is transmitted from one neuron to another.

SYNDROME: Group of symptoms.

SYNERGISM: The joint action of agents so that their combined effect is greater than the algebraic sum of their individual effects.

SYNERGISTIC: Acting together; enhancing the action of another force or agent.

SYNTHESIS: The building up of a chemical compound by the union of its components.

SYSTEMIC CIRCULATION: The general circulation as distinguished from the pulmonary circulation.

TACHY-: Swift, fast.

TACHYPHYLAXIS: Decreased drug effectiveness of the same dose with time.

THEORIZE: To form an opinion based on theory, not actual knowledge.

THEORY: Any hypothesis.

THROMBO-: Clot.

TITRATE: In this context, the balance between amount of drug administered and the expected clinical and/or pharmacophysiologic effect.

TRANS-: Through.

TRANSMEMBRANE: Across a membrane.

TRANSMURAL MI: Entirely through the wall of the heart, from endocardium to myocardial surface; or two-thirds of the way through.

TRANSUDATE: Any substance which has passed through a membrane.

TRANSVENOUS: Transmitted through the veins.

TRI-: Three.

-TROPIC: Toward.

VASCULAR SYSTEM: The blood vessels, including both arterial and venous circulations; most commonly the term is intended to mean the arterial vascular system.

VASOCONSTRICTION: Constriction of the arteries.

VASOPRESSORS: Those agents (sympathomimetic amines) which cause an increase in peripheral resistance (vasoconstriction).

VENESECTION: Same as PHLEBOTOMY.

VENULES: The small veins, particularly those just distal to the capillaries.

VF: Ventricular fibrillation.

VIA: By way of.

VIABLE: Capable of continuing to live.

VISCOSITY: The quality of being viscous to variable degree.

VISCOUS: Sticky or gummy.

VPC: Ventricular premature contraction (PVC).

VT: Ventricular tachycardia.

VULNERABLE PERIOD: The period shown on the ECG during the upsweep of the T-wave or a third of the way down from the apex of the T-wave when an electrical stimulus may initiate ventricular fibrillation.

WT: Weight.

Bibliography

1. Packman, R. C.: *Manual of Medical Therapeutics* (18th ed.; Boston: Little, Brown & Company, 1964).
2. Andreoli, K. G., *et al.: Comprehensive Cardiac Care: A Handbook for Nurses and Other Paramedical Personnel* (St. Louis; C. V. Mosby Company, 1968).
3. Meltzer, L. E., and Kitchell, J. R. (eds.): *The Current Status of Intensive Coronary Care—A Symposium* (Philadelphia: Charles Press, 1966).
4. Wheeler, D. V.; Lillick, L. C., and Kahn, J. M. (eds.): *Aggressive Nursing Management of Acute Myocardial Infarction—A Symposium* (Philadelphia: Charles Press, 1968).
5. Meltzer, L. E.; Pinneo, R., and Kitchell, J. R.: *Intensive Coronary Care: A Manual For Nurses* (Philadelphia: Charles Press, 1965).
6. Meltzer, L. E., and Kitchell, J. R. (eds.): *Cardiac Pacing and Cardioversion—A Symposium* (Philadelphia: Charles Press, 1967).
7. Goodman, L. S., and Gilman, A.: *The Pharmacological Basis of Therapeutics* (3d ed.; New York: Macmillan Company, 1965).
8. White, A.; Handler, P., and Smith, E. L.: *Principles of Biochemistry* (4th ed.; New York: McGraw-Hill Book Company, 1968).
9. Alexander, B., and Wessler, S.: *A Guide to Anti-Coagulant Therapy* (New York: American Heart Association, 1961).
10. *Physicians' Desk Reference—1970* (Oradell, N.J.: Medical Economics).
11. Weil, M. H., and Shubin, H.: Shock following acute myocardial infarction: Current understanding of hemodynamic mechanisms, Prog. Cardiovas. Dis. 11:1, 1968.
12. Katz, A. M.: Effects of interrupted coronary flow upon myocardial metabolism and contractility, Prog. Cardiovas. Dis. 10:450, 1968.
13. James, T. N.: The coronary circulation and conductive system in acute myocardial infarction, Prog. Cardiovas. Dis. 10:410, 1968.
14. Rubin, I. L.; Gross, H., and Arbeit, S. R.: *Treatment of Heart Disease in the Adult* (Philadelphia: Lea & Febiger, 1968).
15. Dac, S., *et al.:* Saving the lives of more M.I. patients in the hospital (Panel Discussion), Patient Care, May, 1968.
16. Dac, S., *et al.:* Saving lives of more M.I. patients the first 45 minutes (Panel Discussion), Patient Care, March, 1968.
17. Austen, W. G., and Morgan, J. M.: Cardiac and peripheral vascular effects of lidocaine and procainamide, Am. J. Cardiol. 16:701, 1965.
18. Conn, R. D.: New drugs for old hearts, Postgrad. Med. 42:71, 1967.
19. Katz, M. J., and Zitnik, R. S.: Direct current shock and lidocaine in treatment of digitalis-induced ventricular tachycardia, Am. J. Cardiol. 18:552, 1966.
20. Thomas, M., and Woodgate, D.: Effect of atropine on bradycardia and hypotension in acute myocardial infarction, Brit. Heart J. 28:409, 1966.
21. Harris, A., and Bluestone, R.: Treatment of slow heart rates following acute myocardial infarction, Brit. Heart J. 28:631, 1966.
22. DeSanctis, R. W.: Electrical conversion of ventricular tachycardia, JAMA 191:96, 1965.
23. Cohn, L. J.; Donoso, E., and Friedberg, C. K.: Ventricular tachycardia, Prog. Cardiovas. Dis. 9:29, 1966.
24. Van Cleve, R. B.: Ventricular tachycardia: Its treatment with emphasis on recent changes in therapy, South. M. J. 60:897, 1967.
25. Smith, J. W.: *Manual of Medical Therapeutics* (19th ed.; Boston: Little, Brown & Company, 1969).
26. Kimball, J. T., and Killip, T.: Aggressive treatment of arrhythmias in acute myocardial infarction: Procedures and results, Prog. Cardiovas. Dis. 10:483, 1968.
27. Lemberg, L.; Castellanos, A., Jr., and Berkovits, B. V.: Pacemaking on demand in AV block, JAMA 191:106, 1965.
28. Staszewska-Barczak, J., and Ceremuzynski, L.: The continuous estimation of catecholamine release in the early stages of myocardial infarction in the dog, Clin. Sc. 34:531, 1968.
29. Harris, C. W., *et al.:* Percutaneous technique for cardiac pacing with platinum-tipped electrode catheter, Am. J. Cardiol. 15:48, 1965.
30. Han, J.; Garcia de Jalon, P. D., and Moe, G. K.: Fibrillation threshold of premature ventricular responses, Circulation Res. 18:18, 1966.
31. Lown, B., *et al.:* Comparative studies of ventricular vulnerability to fibrillation, J. Clin. Invest. 42:953, 1963.
32. Julian, D. G.; Valentine, P. A., and Miller, G. G.: Disturbances of rate, rhythm and conduction in acute myocardial infarction, Am. J. Med. 37:915, 1964.
33. *The Management of Emergencies—The New England Journal of Medicine,* Massachusetts Medical Society, 1966.
34. Gregory, J. J., and Grace, W. J.: The management of sinus bradycardia, nodal rhythm and heart block for the prevention of cardiac arrest in acute myocardial infarction, Prog. Cardiovas. Dis. 10:505, 1968.
35. Friedberg, C. K.; Cohen, H., and Donoso, E.: Advanced heart block as a complication of acute myocardial infarction: Role of pacemaker therapy, Prog. Cardiovas. Dis. 10:466, 1968.
36. Duke, M.: A simple flow chart for use in cardiac arrest, JAMA 202:161, 1967.
37. Lown, B., *et al.:* The coronary care unit: New perspectives and directions, JAMA 199:188, 1967.
38. DeGraff, A. C.: Answers to questions regarding the use and abuse of digitalis, Hosp. Med. 2:18, 1966.

39. Greenspan, K., *et al.*: Countershock, Xylocaine and quinidine in the treatment of digitalis toxicity, J. Indiana M. A. 59:148, 1966.

40. Russell, R. P.; Lindeman, R. D., and Prescott, L. F.: Metabolic and hypotensive effects of ethacrynic acid, JAMA 205:81, 1968.

41. Atkins, L. L.: Experience with furosemide injection, Clin. Med., p. 30, February, 1969.

42. Elek, S. R.: Use of pressor agents in shock following myocardial infarction, Hosp. Med. 4:4, 1968.

43. Davidson, S., and Surawicz, B.: Ectopic beats and atrioventricular conduction disturbances in patients with hypopotassemia, Arch. Int. Med. 120:280, 1967.

44. Spracklen, F. H. N., *et al.*: Use of lignocaine in treatment of cardiac arrhythmias, Brit. M. J. 1:89, 1968.

45. Grossman, J. I., *et al.*: Lidocaine in cardiac arrhythmias, Arch. Int. Med. 121:396, 1968.

46. Weiss, W. A.: Intravenous use of lidocaine for ventricular arrhythmias, J. Internat. Anesth. Res. Soc. 39:369, 1960.

47. Harrison, D. C.; Sprouse, J. H., and Morrow, A. G.: The antiarrhythmic properties of lidocaine and procaine amide, Circulation 28:486, 1963.

48. Gianelly, R., *et al.*: Effect of lidocaine on ventricular arrhythmias in patients with coronary heart disease, New England J. Med. 277:1215, 1967.

49. Klein, S. W.; Sutherland, R. I. L., and Morch, J. E.: Hemodynamic effects of intravenous lidocaine in man, Canad. M. A. J. 99:472, 1968.

50. Jewitt, D. E.; Kishon, Y., and Thomas, M.: Lignocaine in the management of arrhythmias after acute myocardial infarction, Lancet 1:266, 1968.

51. Constantino, R. T.; Crockett, S. E., and Vasko, J. S.: Cardiovascular effects and dose–response relationships of lidocaine, Circulation (supp. II), Vols. 35 & 36, p. 89, October, 1967 (abst.).

52. Lown, B.: In Meltzer and Kitchell.[3]

53. Schumacher, R. R., *et al.*: Hemodynamic effects of lidocaine in patients with heart disease, Circulation 37:956, 1968.

54. Barnett, C. F., Jr.: The use of lidocaine (Xylocaine) in the treatment of cardiac arrhythmias, Delaware M. J. 38:313, 1966.

55. Ettinger, E., *et al.*: Lidocaine in ventricular arrhythmias, Clin. Res. 15:201, 1967.

56. Lewis, K. B.: Treatment of ventricular arrhythmias with intravenous lidocaine (Xylocaine) in non-surgical patients, Clin. Res. 15:213, 1967.

57. Crampton, R. S., and Oriscello, R. G.: Petit and grand mal convulsions during lidocaine hydrochloride treatment of ventricular tachycardia. JAMA 204:109, 1968.

58. Binnion, P. F.: Toxic effects of lignocaine on the circulation, Brit. M. J. 2:470, 1968.

59. Hickam, J. B.; Cargill, W. H., and Golden, A.: Cardiovascular reactions to emotional stimuli: Effect on the cardiac output, arteriovenous oxygen difference, arterial pressure, and peripheral resistance, J. Clin. Invest. 27:290, 1948.

60. Levine, S. A., and Lown, B.: "Armchair" treatment of acute coronary thrombosis, JAMA 148:1365, 1952.

61. Surawicz, B.: Evaluation of treatment of acute myocardial infarction with potassium, glucose and insulin, Prog. Cardiovas. Dis. 10:545, 1968.

62. Thomas, M., *et al.*: Hemodynamic effects of morphine in patients with acute myocardial infarction, Brit. Heart J. 27:863, 1965.

63. Samet, P.: Indications for cardiac pacing in acute myocardial infarction, J. Missouri M. A., September, 1968.

64. Sowton, E.: Cardiac pacemakers and pacing, Mod. Concepts Cardiovas. Dis. 36:31, 1967.

65. Klein, R. F., *et al.*: Catecholamine excretion in myocardial infarction, Arch. Int. Med. 122:476, 1968.

66. Thomas, M.; Malmcrona, R., and Shillingford, J.: Hemodynamic changes in patients with acute myocardial infarction, Circulation 31:811, 1965.

67. Kaplan, J. M., *et al.*: Lupus-like illness precipitated by procainamide hydrochloride, JAMA 192:100, 1965.

68. Sowton, E.: Beta-adrenergic blockade in cardiac infarction, Prog. Cardiovas. Dis. 10:561, 1968.

69. Wessler, S., and Avioli, L. V.: Propranolol therapy in patients with cardiac disease, JAMA 206:357, 1968.

70. Gianelly, R.; Griffin, J. R., and Harrison, D. C.: Propranolol in the treatment and prevention of cardiac arrhythmias, Ann. Int. Med. 66:667, 1967.

71. Friedberg, C. K.: *Diseases of the Heart* (3d ed.; Philadelphia: W. B. Saunders Company, 1966).

72. Marriott, H. J. L.: *Rx for Arrhythmias Handbook* (Oldsmar, Fla.: Tampa Tracings, 1968).

73. Muenster, J. J., *et al.*: Comparison between diazepam and sodium thiopental during DC countershock, JAMA 199:168, 1967.

74. Zoll, P. M., and Linenthal, A. J.: Control of Heart Action by Electrical and Mechanical Means, *Disease-a-Month* (Chicago: Year Book Medical Publishers, Inc., September, 1966).

75. Fearon, R. E.: Comparison of norepinephrine and isoproterenol in experimental coronary shock (observations on the effect of dextran infusion), Am. Heart J. 75:634, 1968.

76. Furman, S., *et al.*: Transvenous pacing: A seven-year review, Am. Heart J. 71:408, 1966.

77. Corday, E., and Irving, D. W.: *Disturbances of Heart Rate, Rhythm and Conduction* (Philadelphia: W. B. Saunders Company, 1961).

78. Wurtman, R. J.: *Catecholamines* (Boston: Little, Brown & Company, 1966).

79. Mittra, B.: Use of potassium, glucose and insulin in the treatment of myocardial infarction, Prog. Cardiovas. Dis. 10:529, 1968.

80. Whalen, R. E., and Saltzman, H. A.: Hyperbaric oxygenation in the treatment of acute myocardial infarction, Prog. Cardiovas. Dis. 10:575, 1968.

81. Lundholm, L.; Mohme-Lundholm, E., and Svedmyr, N.: Catecholamines: Physiological interrelationships, Pharmacol. Rev. 18: 255, 1966.

82. Paine, R.: The nervous system and the heart: I, Missouri Med. 62:663, 1965.

83. Paine, R.: The nervous system and the heart: II, Missouri Med. 62:751, 1965.

84. Paine, R.: The nervous system and the heart: III, Missouri Med. 62:842, 1965.

85. Paine, R.: The nervous system and the heart: IV, Missouri Med. 62:918, 1965.

86. Krasnow, N., *et al.*: Isoproterenol and cardiovascular performance, Am. J. Med. 37:514, 1964.

87. Beregovich, J., *et al.*: Management of acute myocardial infarction complicated by advanced atrioventricular block: Role of artificial pacing, Am. J. Cardiol. 23:54, 1969.

88. Braunwald, E., and Kahler, R. L.: The mechanism of action of cardiac drugs, Physiol. for Physicians 2:1, 1964.

89. O'Rourke, R. A., *et al.*: Lack of effect of procainamide on ventricular function of conscious dogs, Am. J. Cardiol. 23:238, 1969.

90. Udall, J. A.: Drug interference with Warfarin therapy, Am. J. Cardiol. 23:143, 1969 (abst.).

91. Ware, F.: Effects of calcium deficiency and excess on transmembrane potentials in frog heart, Am. J. Physiol. 201:1113, 1961.

92. Anagnostopoulos, L. D., *et al.*: Report of the Committee on Therapeutic Agents on Beta Adrenergic Blocking Agents, Hosp. Formulary Management, p. 28, July, 1968.

93. Abboud, F. M.: Concepts of adrenergic receptors, M. Clin. North America 52:1009, 1968.

94. Jelliffe, R. W.: An improved method of digoxin therapy, Ann. Int. Med. 69:703, 1968.

95. Ende, M.: The pain-relieving properties of pentazocine, A new non-narcotic analgesic, J. Am. Geriatrics Soc. 13:775, 1965.

96. Lal, S.; Chhabra, G. P., and Savidge, R. S.: Cardiovascular and respiratory effects of morphine and pentazocine in patients with myocardial infarction, Lancet 1:379, 1969.

97. DeGraff, A. C.: Axioms in arrhythmia, Hosp. Med. 19, (July), 1967.

98. Cronin, R. F. P.: Effect of isoproterenol and norepinephrine on myocardial function in experimental cardiogenic shock, Am. Heart J. 74:387, 1967.

99. Lyon, A. F., and DeGraff, A. C.: Antiarrhythmic drugs: III. Quinidine toxicity, Am. Heart J. 70:139, 1965.

100. Ruthen, G. C.: Antiarrhythmic drugs: IV. Diphenylhydantoin in cardiac arrhythmias, Am. Heart J. 70:275, 1965.

101. Kayden, H. J.: Antiarrhythmic drugs: V. Pharmacology of procaine amide, Am. Heart J. 70:423, 1965.

102. Kayden, H. J.: Antiarrhythmic drugs: VI. Clinical use of procaine amide, Am. Heart J. 70:567, 1965.

103. Frieden, J.: Antiarrhythmic drugs: VII. Lidocaine as an antiarrhythmic agent, Am. Heart J. 70:713, 1965.

104. Wiedling, S.: *Xylocaine: The Pharmacological Basis of Its Clinical Use* (Stockholm: Almqvist & Wiksell, 1964).

105. Langley, R. B.; Wilson, D. F., and Turner, A. S.: Acute coronary care: A year's experience at Napier Hospital, New Zealand M. J. 67:477, 1968.

106. Sloman, G.; Stannard, M., and Globe, A. J.: Coronary care unit: A review of 300 patients monitored since 1963, Am. Heart J. 75:140, 1968.

107. Dembo, D. H.: Post-resuscitation care after cardiac arrest, Maryland M. J. 15:103, 1966.

108. Meltzer, L. E.; Cohen, H. E., and Wolfgang, S. L.: Sleep regimen for myocardial infarction, Lancet 1:1308, 1968.

109. Booth, S., and Mather, H. G.: Treating coronary thrombosis in an intensive care unit, Nursing Times 64:618, 1968.

110. Kohut, M.: Humanizing coronary care, Chart 65:153, 1968.

111. Jones, B.: Inside the coronary care unit: The patient and his responses, Am. J. Nursing 67:2313, 1967.

112. Rawlings, M. S.: Inside the coronary care unit: Trends in therapeutic management, Am. J. Nursing 67:2321, 1967.

113. New York Heart Association: *Diseases of the Heart and Blood Vessels* (6th ed.; Boston: Little, Brown & Co., 1964).

114. Whalen, R. E., and Starmer, C. F.: Electric shock hazards in clinical cardiology, Mod. Concepts Cardiovas. Dis. 36:7, 1967.

115. Weinberg, S. J.: Electrocardiographic changes produced by localized hypothalamic stimulation, Ann. Int. Med. 53:332, 1960.

116. Folkow, B., and Von Euler, U.S.: Selective activation of noradrenaline and adrenalin producing cells in the cat's adrenal gland by hypothalamic stimulation, Circulation Res. 2:191, 1954.

117. Epstein, E. J., et al.: Artificial pacing by electrode catheter for heart block or asystole complicating acute myocardial infarction, Brit. Heart J. 28:546, 1966.

118. Shapiro, W.: Treatment of postpericardiotomy syndrome, pericarditis of acute myocardial infarction and postinfarction syndrome, Mod. Treatment 4:170, 1967.

119. McIntosh, H. D., and Morris, J. J.: The hemodynamic consequences of arrhythmias, Prog. Cardiovas. Dis. 8:330, 1966.

120. Mainzer, F., and Krause, M.: The influence of fear on the electrocardiogram, Brit. Heart J. 2:221, 1940.

121. Burack, B., and Furman, S.: Transesophageal cardiac pacing, Am. J. Cardiol. 23:469, 1969.

122. Simone, F. A.: Shock, trauma and the physician, New Physician 13:415, 1964.

123. Lillehei, R. C.: Experimental aspects of shock due to hemorrhage, infection, and myocardial failure, New Physician 13:419, 1964.

124. Melby, J. C.: Corticosteroids in shock in man and animals, New Physician 13:426, 1964.

125. Meltzer, L. E.: In Meltzer and Kitchell.[3]

126. Daly, J. W.; Creveling, C. R., and Witkop, B.: The chemorelease of norepinephrine from mouse hearts: Structure-activity relationships; I. Sympathomimetic and related amines. J. Medicinal Chem. 9:273, 1966.

127. Daly, J. W.; Creveling, C. R., and Witkop, B.: The chemorelease of norepinephrine in mouse hearts: Structure-activity relationships; II. Drugs affecting the sympathetic and central nervous systems, J. Medicinal Chem. 9:280, 1966.

128. Epstein, S. E., and Braunwald, E.: Beta-adrenergic receptor blocking drugs, New England J. Med. 275:1106, 1966.

129. Ahlquist, R. P.: Study of adrenotropic receptors, Am. J. Physiol. 153:586, 1948.

130. Dietzman, R. H.; Manax, W. G., and Lillehei, R. C.: Shock: Mechanisms and therapy, Canad. Anaesth. Soc. J. 14:276, 1967.

131. Brady, A. J.: Physiological appraisal of the actions of catecholamines on myocardial contractions, Ann. New York Acad. Sc. 139:661, 1967.

132. Lillehei, R. C., et al.: The nature of irreversible shock: Experimental and clinical observations, Ann. Surg. 160:682, 1964.

133. Block, J. H.; Pierce, C. H., and Lillehei, R. C.: Adrenergic blocking agents in the treatment of shock, Ann. Rev. Med. 17:483, 1966.

134. Dietzman, R. H., and Lillehei, R. C.: The treatment of cardiogenic shock: V. The use of corticosteroids in the treatment of cardiogenic shock, Am. Heart J. 75:136, 1968.

135. Dietzman, R. H., and Lillehei, R. C.: The treatment of cardiogenic shock: IV. The use of phenoxybenzamine and chlorpromazine, Am. Heart J. 75:136, 1968.

136. Smith, H. J., et al.: Hemodynamic studies in cardiogenic shock: Treatment with isoproterenol and metaraminol, Circulation 35:1084, 1967.

137. Bashour, F. A., and Edmonson, R. E.: Silent ventricular tachycardia following acute myocardial infarction, Circulation 32:46, 1965.

138. Brooks, C., et al.: *Excitability of the Heart* (New York: Grune & Stratton, Inc., 1955).

139. Lown, B., et al.: Comparison of alternating current with direct electroshock across closed chest, Am. J. Cardiol. 10:223, 1962.

140. McLean, K. H.; Wynn, A., and Saltups, A.: A coronary care unit: Results of the first year of operation, M. J. Australia 1:471, 1968.

141. Kimball, J. T.; Klein, S. W., and Killip, T.: Cardiac pacing in acute myocardial infarction, Am. J. Cardiol. 19:136, 1967.

142. Roe, B. B.: Intractable Stokes-Adams disease, Am. Heart J. 69:470, 1965.

143. Hall, J. W., III: Steroid therapy in heart-block following myocardial infarction, Lancet 2:1172, 1962.

144. Dall, J. L. C., and Buchanan, J.: Steroid therapy in heart-block following myocardial infarction, Lancet 2:8, 1962.

145. Mittra, B.: Potassium, glucose, and insulin in treatment of heart block after myocardial infarction, Lancet 2:1438, 1966.

146. Kimball, J. T., and Killip, T.: A simple bedside method for transvenous intracardiac pacing, Am. Heart J. 70:35, 1965.

147. Zoll, P. M., and Linenthal, A. S.: A program for Stokes-Adams disease and cardiac arrest, Circulation 27:1, 1963.

148. Prinzmetal, M., and Kennamer, R.: Emergency therapy of cardiac arrhythmias, JAMA 154:1049, 1954.

149. Aber, C. P., and Jones, E. W.: Corticotrophin and corticosteroids in the management of acute and chronic heart block, Brit. Heart J. 27:916, 1965.

150. Sodi-Pallares, D., et al.: Effects of an intravenous infusion of a potassium-glucose-insulin solution on the electrocardiographic signs of myocardial infarction, Am. J. Cardiol. 9:166, 1962.

151. Courter, S. R.; Moffat, J. and Fowler, N.O.: Advanced

atrioventricular block in acute myocardial infarction, Circulation 27:1034, 1963.

152. Paulk, E. A., and Hurst, J. W.: Complete heart block in acute myocardial infarction: A clinical evaluation of intracardiac bipolar catheter pacemaker, Am. J. Cardiol. 17:695, 1966.

153. Chardack, W.: In Meltzer and Kitchell.[3]

154. Zoll, P. M.: In Meltzer and Kitchell.[3]

155. Sowton, E.: In Meltzer and Kitchell.[6]

156. Cohen, H. E.: In Meltzer and Kitchell.[6]

157. Dalle, X. S.: In Meltzer and Kitchell.[6]

158. Kuhn, L. A.: The treatment of cardiogenic shock: I. The nature of cardiogenic shock, Am. Heart J. 74:578, 1967.

159. Kuhn, L. A.: The treatment of cardiogenic shock: II. The use of pressor agents in the treatment of cardiogenic shock, Am. Heart J. 74:725, 1967.

160. Eichna, L. W.: The treatment of cardiogenic shock: III. The use of isoproterenol in cardiogenic shock, Am. Heart J. 74:848, 1967.

161. Uddin, M., and Green, P.: Current status of catecholamines and their implication in various diseases, Manitoba M. Rev. 47:561, 1967.

162. Marriott, H. J. L.: Management of cardiac dysrhythmias complicating acute myocardial infarction, Geriatrics 23:147, 1968.

163. Siddons, H., and Sowton, E.: *Cardiac Pacemakers* (Springfield, Ill.: Charles C Thomas, Publisher, 1967).

164. Deykin, D.: Current concepts: The use of heparin, New England J. Med. 280:937, 1969.

165. Hultgren, H. N., and Flamm, M. D.: Pulmonary edema, Mod. Concepts Cardiovas. Dis. 38:1, 1969.

166. Sulg, I. A., et al.: The effect of intracardial pacemaker therapy on cerebral blood flow and electroencephalogram in patients with complete atrioventricular block, Circulation 39:487, 1969.

167. Ewy, G. A., et al.: Digoxin metabolism in the elderly, Circulation 39:449, 1969.

168. Carvalho, M., et al.: Hemodynamic effects of 3-hydroxytyramine (Dopamine) in experimentally induced shock, Am. J. Cardiol. 123:217, 1969.

169. Gazes, P.: In Meltzer and Kitchell.[3]

170. Foldes, F. F., et al.: Comparison of toxicity of intravenously given local anesthetic agents in man, JAMA 172:1493, 1960.

171. Editorial: Lidocaine in ventricular arrhythmias, Arch. Int. Med. 121:471, 1968.

172. Richmond, D. R.; Mitchell, A. S., and Bernstein, M. B.: Electrical pacing for heart block complicating acute myocardial infarction, M. J. Australia 1:476, 1968.

173. Shillingford, J., and Thomas, M.: Treatment of bradycardia and hypotension syndrome in patients with acute myocardial infarction, Am. Heart J. 75:843, 1968.

174. Lassers, B. W., and Julian, D. G.: Artificial pacing in management of complete heart block complicating acute myocardial infarction, Brit. M. J. 2:142, 1968.

175. Criscitiello, M. G.: Therapy of atrioventricular block, New England J. Med. 279:808, 1968.

176. Dalen, J. E., and Dexter, L.: Pulmonary embolism, JAMA 207:1505, 1969.

177. Januszewicz, W., et al.: Urinary excretion of free norepinephrine and free epinephrine in patients with acute myocardial infarction in relation to its clinical course, Am. Heart J. 76:345, 1968.

178. Friedberg, C. K.: Current status of the treatment of shock complicating acute myocardial infarction, Trauma 9:141, 1969.

179. Gunnar, R. M., et al.: The physiologic basis for treatment of shock associated with myocardial infarction, M. Clin. North America 51:69, 1967.

180. Goldberg, L. I., et al.: The use of Dopamine in the treatment of hypotension and shock after myocardial infarction or cardiac surgery, Am. Heart J. 72:568, 1966.

181. Puri, P. S., and Bing, R. J.: Effect of drugs on myocardial contractility in the intact dog and in experimental myocardial infarction, Am. J. Cardiol. 21:886, 1968.

182. Barrera, F., et al.: Importance of myocardial catecholamines in myocardial infarction, Am. J. M. Sc. 252:177, 1966.

183. Gunnar, R. M., et al.: Ineffectiveness of isoproterenol in shock due to acute myocardial infarction, JAMA 202:1124, 1967.

184. Conn, R. D.: Newer drugs in the treatment of cardiac arrhythmia, M. Clin. North America 51:1223, 1967.

185. Bay, G., et al.: Hemodynamic effects of propranolol in acute myocardial infarction, Brit. M. J. 1:141, 1967.

186. Balcon, R., et al.: A controlled trial of propranolol in acute myocardial infarction, Lancet 2:7470, 1966

187. Clausen, J., et al.: Absence of prophylactic effect of propranolol in myocardial infarction, Lancet 2:920, 1966.

188. Stephen, S. A.: Propranolol in acute myocardial infarction: A multicenter trial, Lancet 2:1435, 1966.

189. Sloman, G., and Stannard, M.: Beta adrenergic blockade and cardiac arrhythmias, Brit. M. J. 4:508, 1967.

190. Wolf, S.: Central autonomic influences on cardiac rate and rhythm, Mod. Concepts Cardiovas. Dis. 38:29, 1969.

191. Editorial: Heparin, New England J. Med. 279:320, 1968.

192. Schmitt, Y.: A program for in-service education in an intensive coronary care unit, Nursing Clin. North America 3:87, 1968.

193. Successful Cardiac Monitoring, Nursing Clin. North America 1:537, 1966.

194. Lown, B., and Shillingford, J.: Symposium on coronary care units: Introduction, Am. J. Cardiol. 20:447, 1967.

195. Day, H. W.: An intensive coronary care area, Dis. Chest. 44:423, 1963.

196. Brown, K. W. G., et al.: An intensive care centre for acute myocardial infarction, Lancet 2:349, 1963.

197. Meltzer, L. E.: Concepts and systems for intensive coronary care, Acad. Med. New Jersey Bull. 10:304, 1964.

198. Killip, T., and Kimball, J. T.: Experience with monitoring myocardial infarction at the New York Hospital-Cornell Medical Center: Comparison of regular hospital care and coronary unit care, Proc. New England Cardiovas. Soc. 24:27, 1965-66.

199. Fakhro, A. M.; Hood, W. B., and Lown, B.: A year's experience with coronary care unit at the Peter Bent Brigham Hospital, Proc. New England Cardiovas. Soc. 24:30, 1965-66.

200. Dorland, W. A. N.: *American Illustrated Medical Dictionary* (24th ed.; Philadelphia: W. B. Saunders Company, 1965).

201. Turner, G. O.: The community approach to reduction of cardiovascular deaths, Missouri Med. 65:746, 1968.

202. Wilburne, M.: The coronary care unit, Hosp. Med., p. 64, February, 1968.

203. Boelling, G. M.: Acute coronary care: An analysis of 196 patients, Missouri Med. 65: 903, 1968.

204. Bailey, R. R., and Beaven, D. W.: A retrospective analysis of 500 patients with acute myocardial infarction, New Zealand M. J. 67:479, 1968.

205. Marshall, R. M.; Blount, S. G., Jr., and Genton, E.: Acute myocardial infarction—Influence of a coronary care unit, Arch. Int. Med. 122:472, 1968.

206. Weinberg, S. L.: The current status of instrumentation systems for the coronary care unit, Prog. Cardiovas. Dis. 11:18, 1968.

207. Killip, T., and Kimball, J. T.: A survey of the coronary care unit: Concept and results, Prog. Cardiovas. Dis. 11:45, 1968.

208. Erwin, G. Y.: Coronary care units in small hospitals, J. M. A. Georgia 57:65, 1968.

209. Fagen, I. D., and Rajagopal, R.: Mortality from myocardial infarction before and after establishment of coronary care units, J. Am. Geriatrics Soc. 16:908, 1968.

210. Lamb, J. D.; McKenney, W. E., and Velis, O. R.: Myocardial infarction and the intensive coronary care unit in a community hospital: Mortality due to arrhythmia can be signi-

ficantly reduced, Rhode Island M. J. 50:329, 1967.

211. Day, H. W.: Effectiveness of an intensive coronary care area, Am. J. Cardiol. 15:51, 1965.

212. Norris, R. M.: Acute coronary care, New Zealand M. J. 67:470, 1968.

213. Paul, O.; Leigh, C. G., and Smyth, G. A.: The patient with a major acute coronary attack and the role of the coronary care unit, Illinois M. J. 132:721, 1967.

214. MacMillan, R. L., et al.: Changing perspectives in coronary care: A five year study, Am. J. Cardiol. 20:451, 1967.

215. Dorph, M.: Coronary care units and the aggressive management of acute myocardial infarction, Delaware M. J. 40:44, 1968.

216. White, B. B.: Survey of acute myocardial infarction over a 4 year period in a community hospital (unpublished).

217. Product Bulletin: Dextran 40 to Enhance Blood Flow in Shock (North Chicago, Ill.: Abbott Laboratories).

218. Rosenberg, A. S., et al.: Bedside transvenous cardiac pacing, Am. Heart J. 77:697, 1969.

219. Jude, J. R., and Elam, J. O.: Fundamentals of Cardiopulmonary Resuscitation (Philadelphia: F. A. Davis Company, 1965).

220. Chazan, J. A.; Stenson, R., and Kurland, G. S.: The acidosis of cardiac arrest, New England J. Med. 278:360, 1968.

221. Massie, E., and Miller, W. C.: The heart size and pulmonary findings during acute coronary thrombosis, Am. J. M. Sc. 206:353, 1943.

222. Keats, A. S., and Telford, J.: Studies of analgesic drugs. VIII. A narcotic antagonist analgesic without psychotomimetic effect, J. Pharmacol. & Exper. Therap. 143:157, 1964.

223. Ad Hoc Committee on Cardiopulmonary Resuscitation: Cardiopulmonary resuscitation, JAMA 198:372, 1966.

224. Surawicz, B.: The role of potassium in cardiovascular therapy, M. Clin. North America 52:1103, 1968.

225. Fisch, C., et al.: Potassium and the monophasic action potential, electrocardiogram, conduction arrhythmias, Prog. Cardiovas. Dis. 8:387, 1966.

226. Surawicz, B., and Lepeschkin, E.: Electrocardiographic pattern of hypopotassemia with and without hypocalcemia, Circulation 8:801, 1953.

227. Surawicz, B., et al.: Quantitative analysis of the electrocardiographic pattern of hypopotassemia, Circulation 16:750, 1957.

228. Lown, B.; Kleiger, R., and Wolff, G.: The technique of cardioversion, Am. Heart J. 67:282, 1964.

229. Shillingford, J. P., and Thomas, M.: Cardiovascular and pulmonary changes in patients with myocardial infarction treated in an intensive care and research unit, Am. J. Cardiol. 20:484, 1967.

230. Pitt, B., and Ross, R. S.: Beta adrenergic blockade in cardiovascular therapy, Mod. Concepts Cardiovas. Dis. 38:47, 1969.

231. Gianelly, R., and Harrison, D. C.: Drugs Used in the Treatment of Cardiac Arrhythmias, Disease-a-Month (Chicago: Year Book Medical Publishers, Inc., Jan., 1969).

232. Bigger, J. T.; Bassett, A. L., and Hoffman, B. F.: Electrophysiological effects of diphenylhydantoin on canine Purkinje fibers, Circulation Res. 22:221, 1968.

233. Scherf, D.: Changes in the electrocardiogram after intravenous administration of diphenylhydantoin sodium (Dilantin) in the acute experiment, Bull. New York M. Coll. 6:82, 1943.

234. Conn, R. D.: Diphenylhydantoin sodium in cardiac arrhythmias, New England J. Med. 272:277, 1965.

235. Helfant, R. H., et al.: Effects of diphenylhydantoin on atrioventricular conduction in man, Circulation 36:686, 1967.

236. Blomgren, S. E., et al.: Antinuclear antibody induced by procainamide: A prospective study, New England J. Med. 281:64, 1969.

237. Pittman, K. A., et al.: Metabolism in vitro and in vivo of pentazocine, Biochem. Pharmacol. 18:1673, 1969.

238. Squire, J. E.: Basic Pharmacology for Nurses (4th ed.; St. Louis: C. V. Mosby Company, 1969).

239. Grossman, J. I.; Cooper, J. A., and Frieden, J.: Cardiovascular effects of infusion of lidocaine on patients with heart disease, Am. J. Cardiol. 24:191, 1969.

240. Silverman, D., et al.: Cerebral death and the electroencephalogram, JAMA 209:1505, 1969.

241. Werk, E. E., Jr., et al.: Interference in the effect of dexamethasone by diphenylhydantoin, New England J. Med. 281:32, 1969.

242. Zipes, D. P.: Treatment of arrhythmias in myocardial infarction, Arch. Int. Med. 124:101, 1969.

243. Rowe, G. G.; Terry, W., and Neblett, I.: Cardiac pacing with an esophageal electrode, Am. J. Cardiol. 24:548, 1969.

244. Church, G., and Biern, R. O.: Intensive coronary care—A practical system for a small hospital without house staff, New England J. Med. 281:1155, 1969.

245. Boyd, D. L., and Williams, J. F., Jr.: The effect of diphenylhydantoin (Dilantin) on the positive inotropic action of ouabain, Am. J. Cardiol. 23:712, 1969.

246. Valencia, A., and Burgess, J. H.: Arterial hypoxemia following acute myocardial infarction, Circulation 40:641, 1969.

247. Hackett, T. P.; Cassem, N. H., and Wishnie, H.A.: The coronary care unit: An appraisal of its psychological hazards, New England J. Med. 279:1365, 1968.

248. Wehrmacher, W. H.: The intensive coronary care unit—A symposium: I, Current M. Digest, p. 853, October, 1969.

249. Danzig, R., and Swan, H. J. C.: Practical experiences in a coronary care unit, Geriatrics, p. 95, June, 1969.

250. Ebert, R. V.: The potential of anticoagulant treatment in acute myocardial infarction, Circulation (supp. IV), vols. 39 & 40, p. 271, November, 1969.

251. Olsen, R. E.: Metabolic interventions in the treatment of infarcting myocardium, Circulation (supp. IV), vols. 39 & 40, p. 195, November, 1969.

252. Hayashi, K. D.; Moss, A. J., and Yu, P. N.: Urinary catecholamine excretion in myocardial infarction, Circulation 40:473, 1969.

253. Corday, E., and Lillehei, R.: Controversies in cardiology: Pressor agents in cardiogenic shock, Am. J. Cardiol. 23:900, 1969.

254. Wehrmacher, W. H.: The intensive coronary care unit—A Symposium: II, Current M. Digest, p. 955, November, 1969.

255. Friedberg, C. K.: General treatment of acute myocardial infarction, Circulation (supp. IV), vols. 39 & 40, p. 252, November, 1969.

256. Swan, H. J. C., et al.: Current status of treatment of power failure of the heart in acute myocardial infarction with drugs and blood volume replacement, Circulation (supp. IV), vols. 39 & 40, p. 277, November, 1969.

257. Grendahl, H., and Sivertssen, E.: Endocardial pacing in acute myocardial infarction, Acta med. scandinav. 186:21, 1969.

258. Koch-Weser, J., et al.: Antiarrhythmic prophylaxis with procainamide in acute myocardial infarction, New England J. Med. 281:1253, 1969.

259. Kleiger, R. E.: Personal communication.

260. Binder, M. J.: Effect of vasopressor drugs on circulatory dynamics in shock following myocardial infarction, Am. J. Cardiol. 16:834, 1965.

261. Soroff, H. S., et al.: Treatment of power failure by means of mechanical assistance, Circulation (supp. IV to Vols. 39 and 40, p. 292), November, 1969.

262. Loeb, H. S., et al.: Hypovolemia in shock due to acute myocardial infarction, Circulation 40:653, 1969.

263. Lown, B.; Kleiger, R., and Williams, J.: Cardioversion and digitalis drugs: Changed threshold to electric shock in digitalized animals, Circulation Res. 17:519, 1965.

264. Kleiger, R., and Lown, B.: Cardioversion and digitalis: II. Clinical studies, Circulation 33:878, 1966.

265. Langhorne, W. H.: The coronary care unit: A year's experience in a community hospital, JAMA 201:662, 1967.

266. Editorial: Oxygen in acute myocardial infarction, Lancet 1:525, 1969.

267. Wilmore, D. W., and Dudrick, S. J.: Safe long-term venous catheterization, Arch. Surg. 98:256, 1969.

268. Corso, J. A.; Agostinelli, R., and Brandriss, M. W.: Maintenance of venous polyethlene catheters to reduce risk of infection, JAMA 210:2075, 1969.

269. Berkowitz, W. D., et al.: The effects of propranolol on cardiac conduction, Circulation 40:855, 1969.

270. Selzer, A., and Wray, H. W.: Quinidine syncope: Paroxysmal ventricular fibrillation occurring during treatment of chronic atrial arrhythmias, Circulation 30:17, 1964.

271. Drug interactions that can affect your patients, Patient Care 1:324, 1967.

272. Ownby, F. D., and Shepard, N. J.: *Advanced Cardiac Nursing,* (Philadelphia: Charles Press, 1970).

273. Langendorf, R., and Pick, A.: Atrioventricular block, type II (Mobitz): Its native and clinical significance, Circulation 38:819, 1968.

Index

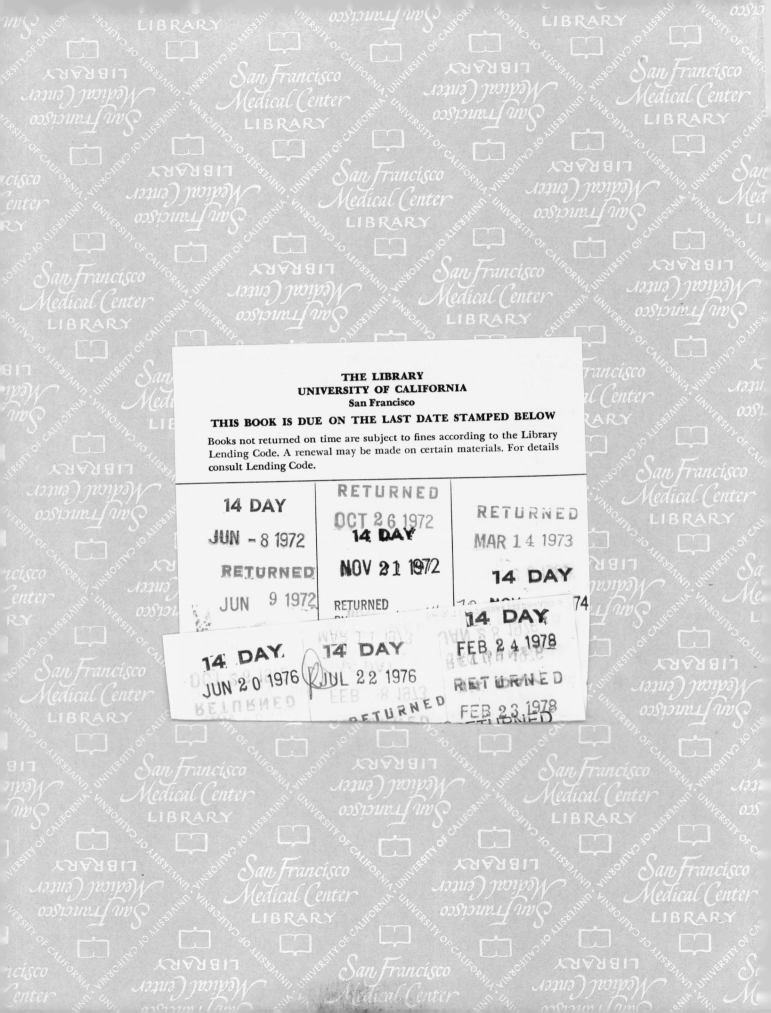